Breast Cancer

Breast Cancer
Thriving Through Treatment to Recovery

Lisa A. Price, ND

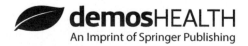

demosHEALTH
An Imprint of Springer Publishing

Visit our website at www.springerpub.com

Demos Health is an imprint of Springer Publishing Company, LLC.

ISBN: 9780826148582
ebook ISBN: 9780826148575

Acquisitions Editor: Beth Barry
Compositor: diacriTech

Medical information provided by Demos Health, in the absence of a visit with a health care professional, must be considered as an educational service only. This book is not designed to replace a physician's independent judgment about the appropriateness or risks of a procedure or therapy for a given patient. Our purpose is to provide you with information that will help you make your own health care decisions.

The information and opinions provided here are believed to be accurate and sound, based on the best judgment available to the authors, editors, and publisher, but readers who fail to consult appropriate health authorities assume the risk of injuries. The publisher is not responsible for errors or omissions. The editors and publisher welcome any reader to report to the publisher any discrepancies or inaccuracies noticed.

Library of Congress Cataloging-in-Publication Data
Names: Price, Lisa A., author.
Title: Breast cancer : thriving through treatment to recovery / Lisa A.Price, ND.
Description: New York : Demos Health, [2019] | Includes bibliographical
   references and index.
Identifiers: LCCN 2019015622| ISBN 9780826148582 | ISBN 9780826148575 (ebook)
Subjects: LCSH: Breast—Cancer—Treatment.
Classification: LCC RC280.B8 P724 2019 | DDC 616.99/44906–dc23
LC record available at https://lccn.loc.gov/2019015622

Contact us to receive discount rates on bulk purchases.
We can also customize our books to meet your needs.
For more information please contact: sales@springerpub.com

Publisher's Note: **New and used products purchased from third-party sellers are not guaranteed for quality, authenticity, or access to any included digital components.**

Printed in the United States of America.
19 20 21 22 23 / 5 4 3 2 1

CONTENTS

This guide is dedicated to all my cancer patients, their families, oncologists, and healthcare team members.

Thanks to the photographers: Food photos, Nicole Barnes Goenner; active lifestyle photos, Nia A. Price-Nascimento.

PREFACE

Truth be told, there is no one magic bullet when it comes to perfect health, treatment, or cures. This is particularly pertinent regarding cancer treatment. While conventional therapies are vital, they result in side effects that can greatly affect quality of life and self-identity and impact recovery and remission. Patients are often told that diet, exercise, and other activities will not make a difference in the development or intensity of symptoms. Nothing could be farther from the truth, and peer-reviewed research supports this. It is therefore of utmost importance that all patients use safe and comprehensive planning during cancer treatment through recovery for best outcomes.

Planning is where this companion guide comes into play. This book is a culmination of my observations of best therapies as a clinician and as a research scientist in complementary and integrative cancer care. I am motivated to share them with you because a holistic approach makes such a positive difference in the lives of patients undergoing cancer treatment through recovery. Besides my own observations, many scientific studies support the effects of specific culinary nutrition, exercise, and mind–body therapies for patients undergoing treatment for breast cancer.

This book will help you understand the various treatments for breast cancer and how they work. I also review the effects of treatment on your immune system and your nutritional status. A diagnosis of cancer often comes with a predictable amount of trauma that can lead to some emotional distress, and I address issues that may result and actions to help mitigate them.

Overall, the book moves from explanations of what is happening to solutions. These are divided into three sections: cookbook (nutrition), exercise, and mind–body therapy, each tailored specifically to benefits for breast cancer patients.

It is my hope that patients engage in a holistic plan that they can incorporate for their lifetime. I highly recommend that you find a qualified and licensed provider to help guide you. If you are having trouble finding a healthcare provider in complementary cancer care with expertise in culinary nutrition, please feel free to contact me at www.drlisapricend.com for an online consult.

May you all be on your path to healing and wellness with hope and strength.

ACKNOWLEDGEMENTS

I would like to thank my parents for catalyzing a deep desire for knowledge, encouraging my curiosity, and for being wonderful examples. Glen, Nia, and Cypress, thank you for understanding my need for time. Finally, to my conventional and naturopathic colleagues, thank you for your endless dedication in supporting all our patients. Thank you, Nicole and Nia, for stepping up to the plate.

Introduction

The greatest thing in the world is to know how to belong to oneself.

—Michel de Montaigne

I have been fortunate to work as a healthcare provider in conventional and private settings around the Puget Sound region, providing a truly integrative approach to treating breast cancer that includes oncologists, radiation oncologists, and other cancer team members. Patients choosing a complementary approach, in my observations, experience fewer side effects, have a better quality of life during treatment, and feel a greater sense of self-control, and thus, self-advocacy. Data shows that they have better outcomes and increased remission rates. Holistic approaches are vital and provide a greater sense of hope and a broader view of patients as whole persons and individuals, not just statistics or numbers.

My work with patients involves guiding them from the start of treatment through recovery and into remission. I dispel myths patients find online, evaluate the safety of supplements relative to conventional therapies they have been prescribed, and direct them to safe and effective therapies appropriate for each individual. Food intake is assessed and specifically modified to reduce or prevent side effects associated with chemotherapy, radiation, or hormone therapy, and patients are encouraged to incorporate consistent exercise and mind–body therapies. Scientific evidence supports the use of holistic approaches indicating increases in remission rates and, certainly, positively affecting quality of life.

I have been inspired and filled with hope the past decade witnessing the power of specific diets and culinary nutrition and use of exercise and mind–body therapies during treatment, especially during breast cancer treatment and beyond. One of my favorite and most inspiring stories follows.

"Liz" came to me when she was initially diagnosed with Stage I triple negative breast cancer. She went through the standard treatment of surgery, chemotherapy (Adriamycin, Cytoxan, and Taxol), and then a round of radiation. She remained NED (No Evidence of Disease) for 9 months before the cancer showed up again. She was again treated but this time with surgery and Taxotere. The cancer continued to grow. At this point, her oncologist told her to get her things in order, there was nothing else he could do. Liz had become quite the self-advocate over time and therefore empowered, and she refused to accept that as the final answer. She searched and pushed to become enrolled in a new clinical trial. The trial disallowed her from using supplements so she turned to culinary nutrition, a specific and individualized diet which I facilitated. As of this writing, she is NED for 18 months (one of the only ones in the trial) and attributes her status to the trial drug and a strict adherence to the diet. She explains her energy level is good, she is sleeping better, and continues to be empowered. Her advocacy now extends to other breast cancer patients, educating patients on the power of food, exercise, and mind–body therapies.

Liz's story illustrates several pearls in the use of complementary therapies and underlines the importance in using a holistic approach during treatment. Patients that develop self-directed safe plans, be it through diet or physical activity, are able to mentally and psychologically improve their quality of lives while undergoing cancer treatment. The second pearl is that these tools do have a physical and physiological effect on the immune system and quality of life.

Complementary therapies include but are not limited to naturopathic medicine, culinary nutrition, acupuncture, and massage therapy. When a holistic approach is managed by an expert team of licensed practitioners in conjunction with conventional therapies, benefits can be achieved for patients.

In the past several years, the rate of remission and stabilization has increased so significantly that a newly recognized phase of treatment has been added called survivorship. With new forms of chemotherapy and immune therapies introduced in the past 10 to 15 years, more people are surviving or living with breast cancer. Patients living with cancer and patients wanting to avoid recurrence need continuing guidance.

The survivor trend was noted by a large and important body of professionals in the cancer world called the Commission on Cancer, a credentialing body composed of surgeons. In 2005, understanding the importance of holistic plans to maintain health, based on peer-reviewed scientific studies, the commission suggested that all accredited cancer institutes create what is known as survivorship programs. These programs provide cancer patients with

- Concise assessment plans with the oncology care team
- Physical needs assessments and services (exercise and physical therapy)
- Nutritional analysis and plans
- Emotional well-being services (mind–body therapies)

Many cancer centers have these services, and you should ask your oncologist or healthcare provider about the survivorship programs she or he is associated with.

Cancer treatment and diagnosis are physically and emotionally traumatic, causing challenges to mental and physical health and to nutritional status. Conventional treatment, which includes surgery, radiation, chemotherapy, and hormone therapy, is effective in treating cancer. However, treatment can, and often does, result in short- and long-term side effects that can affect quality of life and increase the potential risk of long-term ailments including second cancers. Most of the effects are caused by the treatment's direct tissue necrosis or damage, depression of the immune system, and/or nutrient deficiencies.

It is necessary to address these changes for optimal health to be achieved. For example, cancer treatment depletes certain important nutrients. Studies by the National Cancer Institute have found that nutrition, and in particular specific foods, can affect outcome and even help or hurt short- and long-term side effects. Patients receiving nutritional counseling before, during, and after cancer treatment have better outcomes, quality of life, and experience significantly fewer side effects. Furthermore, certain nutrients control the onset of specific side effects from treatment. There are several good studies that validate the importance of nutrition in prevention and remission. One such study, a 2013 survey, demonstrated the need of cancer patients and survivors regarding diet, exercise, and weight management. James-Martin and his team found that patients thought there was a lack of information regarding diet and exercise during and after conventional treatment. As mentioned, those receiving nutritional counseling during and after treatment had better outcomes and reduced side effects. Other holistic interventions also play a significant role in cancer treatment outcomes and prevention of cancer progression.

We know research from the National Cancer Institute and the European Prospective Investigation into Cancer (EPIC) study demonstrates that exercise is the number one factor correlated with remission and cancer prevention. Exercise, both aerobic and resistance training, is important for preventing and decreasing side effects associated with cancer treatment like muscle wasting, fatigue, osteoporosis, and lowered self-esteem. Physical activity can directly affect tumor growth by modulating inflammatory responses in the tumor mass microenvironment. This is an extremely important finding as it relates to recurrence and remission. There are other long-term symptoms that can be addressed by exercise as well. Fatigue, muscle loss, circulation, decreased stamina, and bone loss associated with cancer treatment are simultaneously associated with loss of overall muscle mass. Fatigue associated with muscle loss is in turn associated with increased risk of developing osteopenia and osteoporosis. Hormone treatments using an aromatase inhibitor like Anastrazole put patients at a high risk of developing osteoporosis.

The other reason addressing nutrition, exercise, and emotional needs is important is that these therapies help to decrease *the fear* associated with long-term side effects of cancer treatments, namely chemotherapy, radiation, and hormone therapy. Studies and statistics do show that use of these vital therapies come with long-term risks, including the development of second cancers such as leukemia. The fear of developing side effects during treatment and during recovery is a weight that creates an immense amount of anxiety. Holistic plans can have a positive effect on quality of life and substantially decrease anxiety and worry for cancer patients. In addition, they can return some sense of agency and self-control to patients.

That is why this book is a vital resource for anyone diagnosed with cancer. There is an obvious need for a comprehensive holistic resource for cancer patients, oncologists, and even pharmaceutical companies that addresses minimizing short- and long-term side effects, and therefore the negative association patients have with therapies. This guide provides solutions rather than just highlighting the problematic and burdensome side effects of treatment.

This book is written for cancer patients and their families who would like to use a comprehensive, complementary approach.

Suggestions are based on the general recommendations of the Commission on Cancer and guided by statistical data gathered by the National Cancer Institute to address healing through cancer treatment and beyond. Information presented is supported by hundreds of scientific studies.

This book contains holistic information specific for breast cancer patients that will

- Help you understand your treatment
- Help you understand the possible long- and short-term side effects and provide some solutions to preventing or decreasing them

- Guide you in finding appropriate and safe levels of nutrition via food to use during each treatment phase into recovery (includes 30 recipes)
- Provide you with suggestions for appropriate and safe exercise
- Articulate questions and feelings you might be experiencing throughout treatment and into recovery; and options for therapies that help to restore emotional well-being

ORGANIZATION OF THE BOOK

This book is organized by chapters. Chapters 1 and 2 explain conventional treatments for breast cancer, how they work, and physiological and emotional side effects. The remaining chapters are dedicated to helpful solutions, including nutrition and recipes, exercise, and mind–body therapies.

Within the first chapter, you will find brief descriptions of each treatment type (chemotherapy, radiation, surgery, and hormone therapy), its objective, and its effects on your body. The second chapter focuses on the impact diagnosis has on mental health and how treatment affects your immune system and emotional well-being.

Chapter 3 contains recipes with information related to nutritional content. Chapter 4 focuses on exercise specifically geared to reducing side effects of treatment and promotion of remission. Each exercise is described and includes benefits and a suggested heart rate or goal frequency.

Because there are unique mental health challenges that arise because of diagnosis and treatment, the Chapter 5 is devoted to different mind–body therapies for nurturing emotional well-being. Each suggestion includes a description of the therapy, its goal or purpose, and information on how to contact appropriate professionals in your area. Finally, Chapter 6 summarizes the wholistic plan presented in the guide and offers encouragement on your journey.

The book concludes with a helpful appendix to guide you to professional organizations and resources for further information.

This book is best used throughout the whole duration of treatment, though it is also very beneficial through recovery and during maintenance as well.

As soon as I got the diagnosis, I began to look for what else I could do to help the process. I knew there were things that I could do to help myself through treatment to keep me strong, side effects low and keep cancer from coming back. I changed my diet and started being more selective about what goes into my body. I also started on a regular exercise routine to combat fatigue and also for stress. I became more consistent with my yoga practice. All of these things made a difference, and I continue them all to this very day. They're not prescriptions, but I treat them like that.

—K.C.

CHAPTER 1

Understanding Chemotherapy, Surgery, Radiation, and Hormone Therapy

"Find the seed at the bottom of your heart and bring forth a flower."

—Shigenori Kameoka

Breast cancer, besides skin cancer, is the most common cancer occurring in women, accounting for 12.4% of all new cancer diagnosis. Breast cancer treatment, however, does not fall into a one size fits all. Treatment depends on the extent of and progression of the disease, on the individual, and on other illnesses that the patient might have.

What is for certain is that many women diagnosed with breast cancer will live for many years or decades with cancer, or after being treated for the cancer and declared with No Evidence of Disease! Even more hopeful, biotechnology and immune therapies are moving at light speed ahead. These innovations will enable treatments to be even more effective, less invasive, and more individualized.

Breast cancer patient treatment protocols can fall into several categories based on the location, extent of the disease, hormone receptor status, genetic mutations, age of patient, and other illnesses. In general, there are four different types of treatments:

- Surgery
- Chemotherapy and immunotherapy
- Radiation
- Hormone therapy

So how is it determined which treatment is best for you?

Many clinicians follow standardized protocols for newly diagnosed and reoccurring breast cancer. Treatment protocols may change based on patient response to treatment, genetic mutation status, or progression of the disease. Let us look at the standard treatments used and the objective of each.

SURGERY

Surgery is a local treatment aimed at directly removing the visible tumor mass and exploring the extent of spread in lymph nodes. Most breast cancer patients will have some type of surgery. The exception may be with patients diagnosed with Stage IV metastatic disease, or may depend on the location of the tumor. There are different types of breast surgery that may be done, all with specific objectives:

- *Biopsy.* This is the initial surgery used to determine whether tissue is benign or cancer. Usually one to several tissues are sampled using a needle.

- *Lumpectomy.* This is a breast-conserving surgery where only part of the breast containing the cancer is removed. Patients opting for lumpectomy usually will have to undergo radiation treatment. According to the American Cancer Society (ACS), mastectomies do not give you any better chance of long-term survival or a better outcome from treatment than lumpectomies.

- *Mastectomy.* This surgery involves removing all the breast tissue. This can involve removal of one or both breasts. Patients opting for mastectomies usually do not have to undergo radiation as an additional treatment, but this can vary.

- *Sentinal lymph node dissection/axillary lymph node dissection.* Cancer usually spreads first to lymph nodes under the arm. This surgery removes one to several lymph nodes to determine if and how far the cancer has spread. It is used to determine the extent and type of treatment that will be used.

- *Breast reconstruction.* This surgery usually occurs after chemotherapy and radiation and is meant to restore the shape of the breast. It can involve use of expanders and/or redistribution of abdominal fat in reconstructing the tissue.

Side Effects of Surgery

Surgery and medications given to control pain can cause an array of side effects. The natural response to any tissue damage by the body is inflammation and restoration. The body mobilizes resources such as protein and specific enzymes requiring nutrients to repair the damage. In particular, the body uses vitamins C, E, and B_6, magnesium, and an array of micronutrients.

Drugs given to control pain can create other side effects including severe constipation which can greatly impact quality of life. Other side effects include fatigue, loss of mobility, headaches, neurological pain, and lymphedema.

CHEMOTHERAPY

Chemotherapy is also called a systemic therapy because it affects cells in the entire body. Because cancer cells divide faster and more aggressively, these medications have most of their effect on tumor growth, but also can affect normal cells. Chemotherapy is used to "catch" cancer cells not removed after surgery, or to reduce the size of tumors prior to surgery. Chemotherapy is also used to slow the growth of cancer cells in more advanced cancers.

Chemotherapy works by interfering with the cell's mechanisms for growth and development. There are several different types of medications that all work in different ways. The most common types are

- *Alkylating agents.* These agents affect the cell cycle by creating damage to the DNA and other structures. Patients should proceed with caution when using antioxidants in combination with these therapies. Some commonly used examples falling into this category are Carboplatin, Cisplatin, Oxaliplatin, and Lomustin.
- *Plant alkaloids.* Plant alkaloids were initially discovered and isolated from certain types of plants like periwinkle, the Pacific yew tree, and the Happy Tree. They function by interfering in cell division during various phases. Some commonly used examples include Vincristine, Paclitaxel, Docetaxel, Etoposide, and Irinotecan.
- *Antimetabolites.* These agents mimic naturally occurring substances involved in cell division (RNA and DNA components) and growth. When the agent substitutes itself during the process, cell

division can no longer happen because ultimately the cellular apparatus cannot recognize and use it. They are classified by what substances they mimic. Some examples include Methotrexate, 5-fluorouracil (folic acid), Gemcitabine, and Foxuridine (pyrimidine).

- *Topoisomerase inhibitors.* These therapies interfere with very important enzymes involved in cell division which affects the proper structure of DNA. Some examples include Ironotecan and Etoposide.

- *Immunotherapies.* This category is also known as antitumor antibodies or monoclonal antibodies. They work in a very different way than the previous categories as they are more directed but still have systemic affects. Antibody therapies work by attaching themselves to antigens on the surface of cancer cells or cell receptors. Once they attach, they can recruit other parts of the immune system to destroy these cells. Some commonly used examples include Herceptin and Kadcyla (TDM-1), both used in human epidermal growth factor receptor 2 (HER2) positive patients, Avastin, and Erbitux.

Side Effects of Chemotherapy

Most chemotherapies, including targeted therapies, affect all cells of the body. We call their effect systemic. All more or less act on the ability of cells to divide or involve DNA damage. Normal cells most affected by these affects are mucosal cells, which are any cells along the gastrointestinal tract (e.g., from the mouth to the anus). These cells divide quickly and are most subjected to the action of chemotherapy. Not surprisingly, many of the side effects we see involve gut issues and nutritional deficiencies. Side effects include nausea, loss or alternations in taste, loss of appetite, constipation and/or diarrhea, and fatigue. Other symptoms include hair loss (not all therapies), decreases in red and white blood cells, and problems sleeping.

In general, nutritional deficiencies occurring during chemotherapy include potassium, magnesium, calcium, phosphorus, carnitine, taurine, and glutamine. It is important to note that nutrient deficiencies will vary and be dependent on individual profiles and therapy type. It is important for each patient to be individually assessed by a professional.

RADIATION

Radiation therapy, also known as radiotherapy, is a local targeted treatment which uses high-dose, focused radiation to kill cancer cells. It is used after surgery directly in the area from which the tumor was removed to reduce the risk of recurrence. It is also used directly to kill tumors. In both cases, the objective is to damage the DNA of the cell.

External beam radiation is the most commonly used form. It is targeted and focused. Some radiation oncologists will also use whole breast radiation in certain cases. This treatment involves radiating a larger area of the breast. Tissues that might be treated include breast areas, lymph nodes, and other areas that might be involved in the spread of cancer.

This therapy is effective because cancer cells, unlike normal healthy cells, are not able to effectively repair damage and thus are more prone to death. Radiation does cause damage to normal, healthy cells, but these cells are more resilient and more effective at repairing themselves than cancer cells are.

Radiation treatment is usually a lot faster and more simplistic relative to surgery or chemotherapy treatment. Patient visits usually last no more than 13 to 30 minutes, 5 days a week, for several weeks. This treatment schedule will vary depending on the assessment and recommendations by your oncologist.

Side Effects of Radiation

The most commonly reported side effect from radiation treatment by far is fatigue. The fatigue is cumulative over the several weeks course of treatment. Fatigue may be related to several factors, but two greatly contribute to this side effect. When patients are treated with radiation, there is damage to normal healthy cells as well as cancer cells. The body immediately acts to repair itself, mobilizing needed resources, in particular protein, magnesium, and vitamins like C and B_6.

Daily radiotherapy can also take a psychological toll which can affect energy levels as well. Though treatment is short, daily reminders of a cancer diagnosis can contribute to some transitional depression that may be associated with fatigue.

Other common side effects include skin irritation to burns and armpit irritation followed by decreased range of motion. Radiation travels through layers of epidermis, and thus it is important to treat the affected area daily.

Decreases in white blood cells can occur. Less likely with advanced technology are heart and lung damage.

HORMONE THERAPY

Hormone therapy is also known as selective estrogen degraders and endocrine therapy. It is very different from hormone replacement therapy (HRT) and quite the opposite. With hormone therapy, oncologists are looking to decrease exposure and production of estrogen, while with HRT, estrogen is looked to be increased through taking prescribed hormones.

HRT is a standard option for patients with estrogen-sensitive breast cancer. The objectives are to

- Lower the concentration of hormones in the body
- Block the action of estrogen on breast cancer cells

There are several types of hormone therapies used in treatment of hormone-sensitive breast cancer. These include Tamoxifen, Evista, and Fareston. These are selective estrogen receptor modulators and they block the action of estrogen. Aromatase inhibitors include Arimidex, Aromasin, and Femara. These act to lower the amount of hormone produced by the body.

Side Effects of Hormone Therapy

The objective of hormone therapy is to quickly reduce the production of estrogen or the availability of estrogen in patients with estrogen-sensitive breast cancers. Estrogen plays a protective role for the heart and bones, and plays a slight role as an anti-inflammatory.

Quick withdrawal of estrogen is frequently associated with menopausal symptoms, including the common side effects of hot flashes and night sweats. Mood changes, including depression, can be included into this category as well, in addition to sleep disturbances.

The issue that seems to create the most problematic side effect is joint pain and tenderness. Sometimes this issue becomes such a debilitating problem that women choose to stop treatment rather than stay on it with a severely negative quality of life.

Long-term side effects are osteoporosis and heart disease.

It is important to include diet, supplements, and exercise that support bones and heart function, and which are anti-inflammatory, during hormone therapy treatment. We will take a look at plans in Chapter 3.

NONSTANDARD OPTIONS

In my practice, I have been asked frequently about the validity of nonstandard therapies in the treatment of breast cancer. Because of my conventional training as a biochemist, my answer is always the same: nonstandard options are therapies not supported by rigorous scientific studies and statistics, and therefore involve significant risk, along with lack of guidance when choosing them. One in particular comes up: intravenous (IV) vitamin C therapy.

The National Cancer Institute is monitoring data for IV vitamin C therapy closely. The protocol used for IV vitamin C was developed at the University of Kansas Medical Center in the 1970s. It has long been controversial, and at the writing of this book, while data looks interesting and promising, no standardized protocols, and little evidence of its effectiveness, exist.

Researchers have recently grown interested in preliminary data showing IV vitamin C boosting the effectiveness of other (radiation and chemotherapy) treatments. This nonstandard therapy needs to be thoroughly researched, however.

Oh gosh, I think I was more afraid of the chemotherapy treatment than the cancer, I think. I had a very close friend who was treated, and it was not a pretty sight. I didn't have a very good impression. I asked my oncologists so many questions. I asked them about lots of stuff including nutrition. They didn't know anything about nutrition. I had to find someone to help me with nutrition if I was going to go through with the treatment for my family. I did. I found Dr. Price and she helped me put together a whole plan that addressed a lot of my fears. I did a lot of things. I did okay through treatment. It was much different than what my friend went through. I can't help but to think it was because of what I was doing with food and my diet.

—R.S.

CHAPTER 2

Emotional Aftermath and Effects on the Immune System

I dwell in possibility.

—*Emily Dickinson*

While there are hereditary and environmental factors that increase risk, breast cancer is not selective. I have patients who have never paid attention to their diets and get minimal exercise, to patients who are relatively young, athletic, with no other medical issues. Regardless of who you are or your chosen lifestyle, you are most likely to initially experience some degree of shock, helplessness, and anxiety when told you have cancer. Most people who have been diagnosed with breast cancer experience a sense of loss of control, and bewilderment of where to begin helping themselves. Let us face it, most of us do not plan on developing cancer and thus have not researched treatments, side effects, or other important information to gain an understanding of what to expect. At diagnosis, the cancer learning curve is steep for patients. This lack of knowledge can create a great deal of anxiety, especially for a person who has been independent up to this point in life. For women, the diagnosis causes turmoil as they are usually the organizers, planners, and the nexus or central connection to everything for their families.

When my patient "Mary" first came to see me, she was still in disbelief that she had been diagnosed. Her initial concern was not for herself but was about who was going to take care of everything if she got sick from the treatment or too fatigued to cook, clean, and run errands for the family. This certainly is a common issue that is more or less a part of almost every breast cancer patient's concern.

A cancer diagnosis and standard treatment create predictable physical and emotional disturbances that can affect long- and short-term quality of life, behavior/coping choices, and immune function, which can subsequently affect outcomes and remission.

Women diagnosed with breast cancer face a unique set of emotional issues.

These unique emotional issues include

- Feeling that primary care person is now disabled
- Feelings of loss of independence
- Physical effects of treatment
- Fear of long-term effects of treatment
- Change in self-esteem
- Fear of recurrence

Women can respond in many ways to being diagnosed, treated, and living with breast cancer. They can feel a wide range of emotions. I have some patients that are very emotionally expressive throughout treatment and others that metaphorically hold their breath until therapy is done. All patients could benefit from counseling and other mind–body therapies to help restore mental peace of mind. I have observed that patients who wait until treatment ends to discuss or deal with feelings usually have the most issues with anxiety and depression. It is important to remember that any response to diagnosis is individual and is a normal response. Here are some frequently reported responses:

- *Shock.* When patients are diagnosed, it is common for them to go blank with shock and then to question the results.
- *Grief.* Patients' grief stems from sudden changes to their lives and their bodies with a cancer diagnosis and treatment.
- *Denial.* Even after seeing the test results, some patients will have a period of denial that the results belong to them or are valid or accurate. Sometimes there is even a distrust of the medical system's ability to make the diagnosis.
- *Disappointment.* Some patients blame themselves and search for reasons in their past where they contributed to "causing" their cancer. Others lose faith in their bodies for having "betrayed" them.
- *Anxiety.* Perhaps the most common response is anxiety. Anxiety stems from a fear of the unknown and also the inability to create agency—that is, a sense of self-control over a situation. A cancer diagnosis, treatment, and remission often feels out of the patient's control.
- *Determination.* Some patients immediately direct their attention to what they can do to beat cancer and glide through treatment.

With professional help or direction, these feelings transform, improve, or go away with time. Though it might feel uncomfortable, it is of vital importance that these stressors be recognized and addressed. Stress of this sort has been shown to lead to later presentations of cancer, decreased medical compliance, and increased chance of development of additional illnesses. Increased psychological stress may increase blood levels of epinephrine and norepinephrine, resulting in increased heart rate, blood pressure, and blood sugar levels, which can predispose patients to developing diabetes, metabolic syndrome, and put them at a higher risk of developing cancer or recurrence.

EFFECTS ON YOUR IMMUNE SYSTEM

I prioritize optimizing immune function as my number one focus for all patients that visit me, and therefore stress, external or internal, is quite often the culprit that I seek to tame.

During every first office call, I ask patients what they would like to get out of the appointment with me, and then I verbally compare and complement what my objectives are—to decrease side effects, increase quality of life, and ultimately help the immune system to rebound and optimally function. I cannot stress how important robust immune cells are in fighting cancer.

All immune cells play a role in the fight against cancer, but four in particular must be working well. These cells are natural killer (NK) cells, macrophage, CD8 cells, and T helper 1 cells. Normally, these circulate in every person and remove precancerous and cancer cells. They can be overwhelmed or suppressed by various factors, including external and internal stressors, and even cancer treatment. My plans are always geared to support the immune system during and after cancer treatment to increase quality of life and promote remission.

Let us now take a general look at what happens to the immune system when we are stressed. When we are stressed, one of the main and more significant things that happens is that there is an elevation of the stress hormone cortisol. This is one of the hormones secreted by the adrenal gland involved in the fight or flight mechanism. Other hormones include adrenaline and epinephrine. In the presence of these hormones, especially when these are secreted chronically, the immune system's ability to fight off antigens and cancer is suppressed. Chronic suppression leaves the body not only vulnerable to cancer but also to infection and other disease processes.

Stress can also have an indirect effect on the immune system as a person may use unhealthy behavioral coping strategies to reduce their stress, such as drinking and smoking. These behaviors are extremely common. Alcohol and smoking are known to increase inflammatory processes and use up vital nutrients used by the immune system to function.

Inflammation is necessary for short-term responses to illnesses and injuries in eliminating viruses and initiating healing, but chronic inflammation causes less than optimal functioning of the immune system and increases risk for chronic diseases.

Chronic stress can also activate latent viruses such as those associated with cold sores and shingles. When the immune system is depressed, we see an increase in these chronic viral infections surfacing.

In addition, high and chronic stress levels can cause depression and anxiety, again leading to higher levels of inflammation. Sustained high levels of inflammation lead to an overworked, overtired immune system that cannot properly protect you.

The creation or exacerbation of additional illnesses when you are dealing with cancer puts a burden on your immune system. Psychological stress is involved in altered immune functioning in many diseases. Altered immune function can cause symptoms of both physical and psychological illnesses. For example, in irritable bowel syndrome, high levels of cortisol can create an increase or exacerbation of gastrointestinal symptoms.

Chronic stress has been shown to increase the risk of developing autoimmune diseases like rheumatoid arthritis, lupus, and Sjogren's. People with autoimmune disease also appear to have difficulty balancing immune responses after exposure to stressors.

Overall, the immune system must be tended to achieve the best outcome and remission. Using a variety of therapies to decrease stress works well for most patients.

My identity prior to cancer and treatment was based on my profession and how much I achieved. I was fueled by stress, and compromised so many healthy things, like sleep and exercise because of my lifestyle. I just lived for work. When I slowed down, I realized that I was not living, and I was not happy. That had become my life. I lived in stress 24 hours a day it seemed. After the diagnosis, my condition allowed for me to reflect and feel. It was a scary place to be to feel. It felt awful until it didn't. My whole life is changed now. I feel like I am finally living for me for the first time in a really long time.

—R.T.

CHAPTER 3

Nurturing Through Nutrients: Easy, Flavorful Recipes

It does not matter how slowly you go as long as you do not stop.

—*Confucius*

Now we get to my favorite part of any resource: the solutions! The goals of the recipes in this book are to aid in

- Preventing metabolic syndrome
- Balancing blood sugar levels
- Reducing inflammation

What we know from studies is that patients receiving nutritional counseling before, during, and after cancer treatment have better outcomes, quality of life, and experience significantly fewer side effects.

This chapter is essentially a mini cookbook with recipes helpful during cancer treatment and beyond.

Many of the side effects caused by conventional cancer treatment are rooted in preexisting nutritional deficits and increased nutritional needs caused by therapies. Common nutritional deficiencies include magnesium, calcium, potassium, and sodium. A deficiency in magnesium, for example, can create or exacerbate elevated or depressed blood pressure, muscle cramps, sleep disorders, or problems with metabolism. Another common side effect of all therapies is fatigue. Fatigue in patients results from an increased turnover of protein, increased nutrient demand for repair, and disturbances associated with fatty acid metabolism. Proper protein supplementation can substantially decrease treatment-related fatigue and tissue recovery.

Recent research studies have determined that nutrition matters during and after treatment. Therapeutic foods can decrease the side effects of conventional cancer treatment, increase quality of life, and increase remission chances. Knowledge of those foods having negative interactions is also vital.

A LITTLE HOUSEKEEPING

The recipes in this book are made with ingredients that are anti-inflammatory, have a low glycemic index, and are nutrient/mineral dense. And they are delicious! When applying my culinary nutrition expertise during cancer treatment, my goal is to help patients achieve an 80% compliance rate with their diet choices. Some things that I have learned:

1. People are tied closely to their tastes and habits with food

2. Small, reasonable changes to diet work better than grand sweeping changes

3. Taste and texture matter; and it especially matters during cancer treatment

In other words, do not "mess" with food unless recipes are going to be flavorful, something recognizable, and easy to make. The good news is that cooking with anti-inflammatory ingredients can encompass all these goals easily. For the most part, and this is thanks to the abundance of different types of food on the planet, many of us already have incorporated eating in a healthy and helpful fashion during cancer care.

Understanding why it is important to eat an anti-inflammatory diet is helpful to compliance. The National Cancer Institute continuously updates its database on several aspects affecting cancer remission and prevention. Many of these recommendations are specific, like reducing intake of red meat to three servings per week. These findings and others are based on nutritional contents of foods that we consume and their inflammatory affects. For example, both cow dairy and red meat contain a higher amount of something called omega 9 fatty acids. These are not "bad" fats per se, but if we consume too many of them, we can tip the balance toward inflammation in our bodies. Inflammation can create damage and reactions that beget more inflammation, causing the cycle to continue. When the damage caused by inflammation exceeds the body's ability to "clean" it up, we begin to get damage at a cellular level. Damaged cells can turn into cancer.

Another example of the importance of eating an anti-inflammatory whole foods diet has to do with insulin sensitivity. Many people mistakenly attribute sugar as being the culprit in feeding cancer cells. This belief is not entirely correct. It is the insulin surges that are related to some solid tumors' aggressive growth. Insulin is a hormone that is secreted in response to glucose, or sugar, levels in the bloodstream. Insulin presence signals to the cells to grow and divide. Normal cells consume the glucose at a normal rate, divide, and then have a mechanism to turn themselves off. Some solid tumor cells, research shows, more aggressively take up glucose, given the signal by insulin, and they do not contain the mechanism to turn off growth or slow down growth. Eating a diet containing complex carbohydrates and whole foods causes the blood sugar and insulin levels to maintain a steady state, that is, no big ups or downs in insulin. Eating this way with whole foods is the foundation of an anti-inflammatory diet.

The easiest way to adhere to an anti-inflammatory diet is first to be conscious of what you are eating. Take a week or two to just assess what you are eating:

- How many boxed and processed foods am I eating?
- How many times a week am I eating out and what kinds of foods am I eating?
- How much processed sugar and simple carbohydrates am I eating per day?
- How many whole foods do I have in my diet?

Once you have assessed what you are eating make steps to trade out one thing at a time. For example, maybe you eat lunch out at a fast food restaurant five times a week. The first step could be that you eat out four times a week and bring a healthy meal from home once per week. Or you could choose to eat at a healthier venue that offers lean meat, salads, and healthy soup options. Small changes, for many, add up to long-term compliance. Of course, some people are very successful in making a 180-degree change in their diet once diagnosed with cancer. That is okay as well.

SUGGESTIONS FOR YOUR PANTRY

I would suggest over time decreasing or eliminating the following foods from your pantry and refrigerator:

Wheat flour	Corn
Corn meal	Soy oil
White sugar	Canola oil
Brown sugar	Cow milk and cheeses
Agave syrup	Soda
Margarine	Fruit juice
White potatoes	Alcohol

Think about replacing them with:

Barley flour	Butter or ghee
Almond flour	Vinegar
Oat flour	Herbs and spices (e.g., rosemary,
Ground flaxseeds	cumin, ginger)
Goat cheese	Extra virgin olive oil
Sheep cheese	Coconut oil
	Walnuts

These foods are readily available at most grocery stores. In addition, you can find them online and at local co-ops and natural food stores.

Wherever you are in the process of dietary changes, know that diet and nutrition do make a difference in treatment side effects and outcome. An anti-inflammatory diet can make a difference, and you can still enjoy your meals with the side benefits increased energy and health protection.

Use these recipes as starting points. Add a side dish or two to one of your favorite meals. Try to integrate slowly so it is not quite a jolt to your regular patterns. For more recipe ideas, check out my blog at www.drlisapricend.com and my Instagram account at @culinarydoc

NUTRITION TIPS PRIOR TO CHEMOTHERAPY TREATMENT

Included here are a few tips that I give to my patients to get through chemotherapy treatments a little better:

- Drink 1 cup of bone broth or vegetable broth daily. Many chemotherapies are depleting in major minerals, deficiencies that can either produce or exacerbate side effects. Bone broth is an excellent way to replenish. Drink this throughout the entire period of treatment even when you are not getting an infusion.

- During infusion, drink 8 to 16 ounces of cold coconut water. The cold of the drink will help to protect your mouth and taste buds, thus decreasing loss of taste, as well as helping to decrease mouth sores. Coconut water also contains a good amount of potassium and other wonderful electrolytes.

- Prior to infusion, make sure you have a breakfast with a good amount of protein with good fats before treatment. Protein and good fats will help your blood sugar level and somewhat counteract the effects that steroids have on it. This will help to decrease nausea and fatigue.

Let us dive into the nitty-gritty and start making meal plans, shall we?

I was one of those people who went from fad diet to fad diet to lose weight to look a certain way. I had been doing it my whole life. Most of those diets were real food in the recent past, but they were still restrictive. When I was diagnosed with cancer, I actually didn't know what kind of diet to use. So, I needed help. Dr. Price recommended using an anti-inflammatory, therapy-based diet based on my individual body. We used a variety of whole foods but focused on food that contained nutrients I'd be prone to depletion by my treatment. What ended up happening was I relearned to eat. I actually stopped being afraid of eating food. It was amazing. Food is medicine.

—S.C.

MORNING DISHES

BREAKFAST HASH

Why not try something different for breakfast than the usual cereal, eggs, and bacon? Fragrant vegetable hash is an excellent way to start your day. This recipe contains aromatic and warming spices and vegetables and includes a lean protein that blends well with the medley. Your gut will love you for it.

NUTRITIONAL ANALYSIS PER SERVING:

Calories—274.7	Sugar—4.4 g	Vitamin D—0.1 IU
Fat—18.4 g	Protein—17.3 g	Vitamin E—3.3 IU
Sodium—100.5 mg	Vitamin A—33.4 mg	Folate—97.9 mcg
Potassium—816.6 mg	Vitamin C—106.0 mg	Vitamin B_6—0.4 mg
Carbohydrates—12.5 g	Calcium—75.5 mg	Vitamin B_{12}—1.2 mcg
Fiber—5.1 g	Iron—2.8 mg	

Makes 2 servings

Ingredients:

1 cup brussels sprouts, minced

1 cup cauliflower, chopped

1 cup broccoli, chopped

½ cup fennel root, fresh, chopped

½ tsp cardamom, dried spice

½ tsp turmeric, dried spice

3 to 4 ounces of ground bison or free-range beef

Olive oil

Salt

Pepper

Directions:

To a pan, add about 2 tbs of olive oil. Heat over medium to high heat and add vegetables and spices. Sauté for 15 minutes, stirring occasionally until soft. Add meat, mix and cook until browned. Salt and pepper to taste.

Nutritional Tip 101: Cauliflower and brussels sprouts belong to a group called cruciferous vegetables. These plants contain chemicals like diindolymenthane that are helpful in modulating estrogen via the liver.

WARM AND SAVORY BREAKFAST WRAPS

Wraps for breakfast are a quick and easy way to make sure you are getting your nutrition at the top of the day. These pack well and are delicious.

NUTRITIONAL ANALYSIS PER SERVING:

Calories—569	Sugar—7.9 g	Vitamin D—1.3 IU
Fat—48.6 g	Protein—15.5 g	Vitamin E—9.7 IU
Sodium—138.9 mg	Vitamin A—313 mg	Folate—165 mcg
Potassium—785.8 mg	Vitamin C—111 mg	Vitamin B_6—0.7 mg
Carbohydrates—23 g	Calcium—93 mg	Vitamin B_{12}—1.6 mcg
Fiber—7.6 g	Iron—2.6 mg	

Makes 1 serving

Ingredients:

1 rice wrap or 1 wilted collard green (blanch green in hot water)

2 eggs

⅓ avocado

½ cup onions

1 tbs garlic

½ cup red pepper

½ tsp turmeric, fresh root, shredded

Extra virgin olive oil

Optional: ¼ Red bell pepper, sliced

Directions:

To a pan, add 2 tbs of olive oil. Heat pan over medium to high heat. Scramble two eggs and add fresh turmeric, onions, garlic, and red pepper. Layer egg on wrap. On top of the egg, add avocado. You may add your red bell pepper strips. Fold wrap like a tortilla. Enjoy.

Nutrition Tip 101: Turmeric contains curcumin, a chemical that is helpful as an anti-inflammatory and in pain reduction.

BASIL-ED EGGS AND YAMS

This dish makes for a hearty breakfast. The yams add some sweetness and texture to the scrambled eggs. Of course, you can never go wrong with adding fresh basil to almost anything.

NUTRITIONAL ANALYSIS PER SERVING:

Calories—358	Sugar—1.2 g	Vitamin D—80 IU
Fat—24 g	Protein—14 g	Vitamin E—5 IU
Sodium—133 mg	Vitamin A—224 mg	Folate—79 mcg
Potassium—774 mg	Vitamin C—16 mg	Vitamin B_6—0.4 mg
Carbohydrates—24 g	Calcium—84 mg	Vitamin B_{12}—1.6 mcg
Fiber—3.3 g	Iron—2.3 mg	

Makes 2 servings

Ingredients:

4 eggs

½ cup basil, fresh

1 cup yams, cubed

1 tsp turmeric, powder

1 to 2 tbs garlic, minced

2 to 3 tbs extra virgin olive oil

Salt

Pepper

Directions:

Preheat oven to 400°.

Cube yams into ½- to 1-inch squares. In a bowl, combine 1 tbs of oil, turmeric, minced garlic, and salt. Roast the yams for 20 to 30 minutes or until soft.

Place the eggs in a bowl and whisk them until even. Add basil and continue whisking.

To pan, add olive oil and bring pan to a medium to high heat. Add the roasted yam mixture and sauté for 3 to 4 minutes. Add egg mixture and scramble all ingredients together. Cook eggs until done (no runny areas). Add salt and pepper to taste.

Nutrition Tip 101: Sweet potatoes contain a rich source of fiber. They also contain minerals, such as calcium, selenium, and iron, and the B vitamins.

BREAKFAST IN A JAR

This breakfast is not only fast it's delicious and never gets old. By using a variety of spices and nuts you can change the flavor and texture. You can serve it hot or cold. This recipe is very versatile and provides a great source of soluble fiber.

NUTRITIONAL ANALYSIS PER SERVING:

Calories—369	Sugar—18.4 g	Vitamin D—0 IU
Fat—22.1 g	Protein—7.4 g	Vitamin E—0.7 IU
Sodium—13.8 mg	Vitamin A—1.9 mg	Folate—27.9 mcg
Potassium—522 mg	Vitamin C—1.8 mg	Vitamin B_6—0.1 mg
Carbohydrates—41 g	Calcium—75.9 mg	Vitamin B_{12}—0 mcg
Fiber—8.2 g	Iron—3.7 mg	

Makes 1 serving

Ingredients:

¼ cup uncooked oatmeal

½ tsp sesame seeds

½ tsp chia seeds

½ tsp flaxseeds, ground

½ tsp cinnamon

1 tbs dried dates

1 tbs cashews

Coconut milk

Directions:

To a mason jar, add oatmeal and all other dry ingredients, including cinnamon. Mix by putting the lid on the jar and shaking. Before going to bed, add coconut milk to an inch above the ingredients. Place in refrigerator until morning. You can eat it cold or heat it up. Enjoy.

Nutrition Tip 101: Chia seeds contain a good amount of soluble fiber which benefits gut health. In addition, chia seeds also have a good amount of protein.

COCOA AND CHIA PUDDING

There's no shame in starting your day out with chocolate, as long as that meal contains a wonderful variety of healthful nutrients and low sugar content. This pudding is smooth, creamy, and very satisfying.

NUTRITIONAL ANALYSIS PER SERVING:

Calories—407	Sugar—3.9 g	Vitamin D—0.5 IU
Fat—33.7 g	Protein—11 g	Vitamin E—7.8 IU
Sodium—36.1 mg	Vitamin A—32 mg	Folate—124.4 mcg
Potassium—836 mg	Vitamin C—10 mg	Vitamin B_6—0.4 mg
Carbohydrates—28 g	Calcium—213.6 mg	Vitamin B_{12}—0.2 mcg
Fiber—17 g	Iron—3.4 mg	

Makes 1 serving

Ingredients:

½ avocado

1 tbs chia seeds

1 tbs flaxseeds, ground

2 tbs walnuts

1 tbs cocoa, powdered

1 tsp dried dates

¼ cup coconut or hemp milk (vanilla or plain)

Optional: ½ tsp of vanilla extract

Directions:

To the coconut milk (or hemp), add the dates, chia seeds, and ground flaxseeds. Let sit overnight or for 30 to 50 minutes in the refrigerator. You can use an 8-ounce mason jar. Add this mixture to a blender along with the avocado, cocoa, and walnuts. You may add the vanilla extract here. Blend. Enjoy.

Nutrition Tips 101: Cocoa powder contains a good amount of magnesium, which is a nutrient that is commonly deficient during cancer treatment.

MAIN DISHES

LASAGNA (OPTION: GROUND TURKEY)

Some recipes were meant to be mostly comfort and this is one of them, but with a healthy twist. This vegetarian lasagna blends Italian spices well with goat and feta cheeses. It is lighter than conventional lasagna but will leave you completely satisfied.

NUTRITIONAL ANALYSIS PER SERVING:

Calories—570

Fat—33 g

Sodium—410.1 mg

Potassium—2032.6 mg

Carbohydrates—47.1 g

Fiber—10.1 g

Sugar—14.1 g

Protein—31.1 g

Vitamin A—896.9 mg

Vitamin C—165.1 mg

Calcium—753.0 mg

Iron—5.5 mg

Vitamin D—0.8 IU

Vitamin E—4.0 IU

Folate—183.1 mcg

Vitamin B_6—1.3 mg

Vitamin B_{12}—0.5 mcg

Makes 4 servings

Ingredients:

5 zucchinis, medium to large, sliced, ¼-inch thick

8 ounces goat cheese, hard

1 egg

⅓ cup oat milk

¼ cup basil, fresh, chopped

1 tsp thyme, fresh

1 tsp oregano, fresh

⅓ cup of feta, grated

3 garlic cloves

1 bunch kale, deveined, thinly sliced

2 cups shiitake mushrooms, sliced

Pasta sauce, premade

2 tbs extra virgin olive oil

Salt

Directions:

Preheat oven to 375°.

Lay sliced zucchini slices on a plate and sprinkle with a pinch of salt on both sides. Leave on plate in a single layer (not piled on top of each other) for about 30 minutes. Pat the zucchini dry with a paper towel.

In a bowl, combine and mix egg, goat cheese, oat milk, basil, and all other spices except for garlic. Set aside. To a pan, add 2 tablespoons of olive oil over medium high heat. Sauté kale, mushrooms, and minced garlic until kale is limp. Place mixture into a separate bowl.

If you are using ground turkey, brown the meat at this point and also add it to its own separate bowl.

In a casserole dish (9 × 13 inches), begin layering with zucchini slices. Cover the bottom. Add a thin layer of the goat cheese mix, followed by a layer of pasta sauce. Add the kale–mushroom mix on top of the pasta sauce. Add a turkey layer if you chose this option. Repeat the layering. The last layer of the lasagna should be zucchini with some pasta sauce. Add a single layer of shredded goat cheese on top.

Place in the oven for 35 to 40 minutes. Remove from oven and let cool for 15 to 20 minutes.

Enjoy.

Nutrition Tip 101: According to the National Cancer Institute, cow dairy should be limited to no more than four servings per week. Goat and feta (sheep) cheeses are best choices when indulging because of their higher content of omega 3 fatty acids.

FALL LENTIL STEW

This dish is a hearty plant-based stew. You'll love the variety of textures and flavors that you find in this savory recipe. The best part is the ease of making such a delicious meal.

NUTRITIONAL ANALYSIS PER SERVING:

Calories—445	Sugar—8.5 g	Vitamin D—0 IU
Fat—1.4 g	Protein—28.0 g	Vitamin E—5.5 IU
Sodium—101.2 mg	Vitamin A—1011 mg	Folate—507.1 mcg
Potassium—1503.8 mg	Vitamin C—50.7 mg	Vitamin B_6—1 mg
Carbohydrates—81.8 g	Calcium—125.9 mg	Vitamin B_{12}—0 mcg
Fiber—14.9 g	Iron—8.3 mg	

Makes 4 servings

Ingredients:

1 cup uncooked lentils, 3 cups water	1 sweet potato, medium, cubed
3 to 4 garlic cloves	½ tsp cardamom
1 cup carrots, chopped	½ tsp turmeric
1 cup broccoli florets, chopped	Salt to taste

Directions:

To a large pot, add water and lentils. Bring to a boil over high heat and then reduce to medium. Cook the lentils for about 30 to 40 minutes before adding the rest of the ingredients. Add ingredients and cook an additional 30 to 40 minutes over low to medium heat. If the stew thickens too much, add additional water.

Nutrition Tip 101: Lentils contain a good amount of plant-based protein, and they are much easier to digest than many beans. They contain a very good amount of folate.

LIME HALIBUT WITH ROASTED CAULIFLOWER

This recipe has a perfect blend of lean protein and spices. It is savory and bright. The cauliflower adds a crispiness to the texture of the overall meal.

NUTRITIONAL ANALYSIS PER SERVING:

Calories—526	Sugar—10.5 g	Vitamin D—4.2 IU
Fat—44.8 g	Protein—35.8 g	Vitamin E—8.4 IU
Sodium—216.3 mg	Vitamin A—358.9 mg	Folate—298 mcg
Potassium—2198 mg	Vitamin C—287 mg	Vitamin B_6—0.9 mg
Carbohydrates—30.1 g	Calcium—256 mg	Vitamin B_{12}—1.2 mcg
Fiber—10.1 g	Iron—7.4 mg	

Makes 2 servings

Ingredients:

8 ounces halibut

1 can coconut milk

1 lime, juice from

1 cup fresh parsley

1 cup fresh cilantro

3 cups cauliflower, chopped

2 tbs extra virgin olive oil

½ tsp turmeric, dried

Salt to taste

Directions:

Heat oven to 400°.

Place fresh halibut fillet in a cast iron pan or other cookware that is oven safe. In a separate bowl, mix the cauliflower, olive oil, and the turmeric. Try to coat the cauliflower with the spice. Place mixture in the pan with the fish. Cauliflower should be on the sides of the fish rather than directly on it.

In a blender, combine coconut milk, cilantro, parsley, and juice from the lime. Mix on high setting Pour mixture over fish and also cauliflower. Cook in oven for 20 to 30 minutes or until fish is flaky.

Nutrition Tip 101: Parsley contains a good amount of selenium, a mineral that acts as an antioxidant. It also contains another antioxidant called apigenin that is helpful in cellular repair.

ORANGE BROCCOLI WITH CASHEWS AND BASIL OVER WILD RICE

What a bright and sunny side dish this is as a stand-alone vegetable side dish or over wild rice. The combination of ginger and garlic adds some warmth, while the cashews and orange flavor add naturally sweet overtones.

NUTRITIONAL ANALYSIS PER SERVING:

Calories—186.3	Sugar—4.6 g	Vitamin D—0 IU
Fat—14.6 g	Protein—4.3 g	Vitamin E—2.5 IU
Sodium—163.9 mg	Vitamin A—37.4 mg	Folate—73.1 mcg
Potassium—405.1 mg	Vitamin C—94.5 mg	Vitamin B_6—0.2 mg
Carbohydrates—12.3 g	Calcium—54.2 mg	Vitamin B_{12}—0 mcg
Fiber—2.5 g	Iron—1.4 mg	

Makes 4 servings

Ingredients:

½ cup orange juice

1 tbs tamari

¼ tbs fresh ginger, grated

¼ tbs garlic, minced

1 tbs sesame seed oil

4 cups broccoli, florets, chopped

¼ cup cashews

¼ cup basil, fresh, chopped

2 to 4 tbs of avocado oil

Directions:

In a pan over medium to high heat, add 2 tablespoons of avocado oil and broccoli. Sauté for 5 minutes. In a separate bowl, mix the orange juice, tamari, garlic, and ginger. After 5 minutes of the broccoli cooking, add the mixture and cook for another 5 to 10 minutes. Remove from heat. Add basil, sesame oil, and cashews. Toss. Cover and let sit for 5 minutes. Serve warm. Enjoy.

Nutrition Tip 101: Ginger is an excellent spice to help with nausea and inflammation.

LIMA BEAN SOUP WITH BACON AND FETA

I have to admit that this soup is another comfort food altered to be more healthful while maintaining the flavor. Lima bean soup is savory and creamy. Including a small amount of bacon and feta cheese to the soup adds a nice amount of saltiness one might crave.

NUTRITIONAL ANALYSIS PER SERVING:

Calories—272	Sugar—4.5 g	Vitamin D—0.1 IU
Fat—13.6 g	Protein—11.1 g	Vitamin E—0.7 IU
Sodium—366.6 mg	Vitamin A—389 mg	Folate—69.8 mcg
Potassium—748.4 mg	Vitamin C—35 mg	Vitamin B_6—0.4 mg
Carbohydrates—27.7 g	Calcium—217.3 mg	Vitamin B_{12}—0.5 mcg
Fiber—9.2 g	Iron—3.6 mg	

Makes 4 servings

Ingredients:

2 cups lima beans, uncooked

4 cups of water

1 cup parsley, fresh, chopped

½ cup dill, fresh

1 cup carrots, chopped

½ cup green onions, chopped

2 tbs garlic, minced

1 tbs turmeric, fresh

2 slices of bacon, organic beef or turkey

4 ounces feta cheese

Directions:

To a large pot, add water and beans. Turn heat to medium high. Cook for 20 to 30 minutes. Turn heat to low to medium and add dill, carrots, onions, garlic, turmeric, and bacon. Mix in and cook for 20 more minutes. Crumble 1 ounce of feta per serving. Enjoy.

Nutrition Tip 101: Lima beans contain an excellent source of potassium, a common nutrient which is deficient during cancer treatment.

ACORN SOUP WITH A KICK

This is my favorite soup. It is easy to make, requiring only three steps, and has a fantastic flavor with some heat created by lemongrass, cilantro, and jalapeno pepper. The heat is mellowed out a bit by the coconut milk used in the recipe. Truly a delicious soup.

NUTRITIONAL ANALYSIS PER SERVING:

Calories—166.9	Sugar—1.6 g	Vitamin D—0 IU
Fat—9.4 g	Protein—3.4 g	Vitamin E—0.9 IU
Sodium—110.2 mg	Vitamin A—112.7 mg	Folate—54.9 mcg
Potassium—845.4 mg	Vitamin C—25.3 mg	Vitamin B_6—0.3 mg
Carbohydrates—21.6 g	Calcium—85.3 mg	Vitamin B_{12}—0 mcg
Fiber—3.7 g	Iron—3.0 mg	

Makes 6 servings

Ingredients:

2 acorn squash

16 ounces coconut milk

16 ounces of vegetable broth

1 bunch cilantro

½ fresh jalapeno pepper

¼ tsp habanero pepper, dry

6 cloves garlic

2 tbs roasted chili paste

2 stalks of lemon grass
(approximately 3–4 inches long)

1 tbs of salt (or to taste)

Directions:

Steam acorn squash in a covered pot with about 1 inch of water until soft (about 10–15 minutes on high heat). Remove and scrape out seeds to discard. Continue scraping out the squash flesth and place it in a blender.

Add all other ingredients to the blender. Blend until uniform in color (about 3 minutes). Pour the mixture into a pot and simmer for 20 to 30 minutes. The spiciness of this soup can be adjusted by adding more or less of the habanero pepper spice.

Nutrition Tip 101: Squash contains a great amount of soluble fiber which is beneficial for gut health, including normal bowel function. In addition, many squashes contain good amounts of vitamin A and beta-carotene.

LENTIL SALAD WITH PARSLEY, MINT, AND LIME

This salad is a light, refreshing meal and is quick to prepare. It stores well in the refrigerator for three days and travels easily.

NUTRITIONAL ANALYSIS PER SERVING:

Calories—265.2	Sugar—6.0 g	Vitamin D—0 IU
Fat—1.2 g	Protein—19.7 g	Vitamin E—1.3 IU
Sodium—26.6 mg	Vitamin A—204.9 mg	Folate—439.3 mcg
Potassium—1067 mg	Vitamin C—99.5 mg	Vitamin B_6—0.5 mg
Carbohydrates—47.3 g	Calcium—108.5 mg	Vitamin B_{12}—0 mcg
Fiber—10.9 g	Iron—9.2 mg	

Makes 2 servings

Ingredients:

2 cups lentils, cooked

1 cup parsley, chopped

½ cup mint, fresh, chopped

1 lime, juiced

½ cup red pepper, chopped

¼ cup green onions, chopped

Salt

Directions:

In a large bowl, combine all solid ingredients. Add the lime juice last and toss. Enjoy.

Nutrition Tip 101: Mint is a carminative, meaning that it is helpful with gas and upset stomachs.

BLACK BEAN SALAD

What a variety of textures and flavors this salad provides! When you start eating this meal, you'll be surprised by the unexpected textures and flavors that go into this recipe.

NUTRITIONAL ANALYSIS PER SERVING:

Calories—264	Sugar—2.7 g	Vitamin D—0 IU
Fat—12.9 g	Protein—10.3 g	Vitamin E 3.6 IU
Sodium—16.8 mg	Vitamin A—87.6 mg	Folate—199.4 mcg
Potassium—814.9 mg	Vitamin C—19.8 mg	Vitamin B_6—0.1 mg
Carbohydrates—30.4 g	Calcium—54.8 mg	Vitamin B_{12}—0 mcg
Fiber—11.1 g	Iron—2.8 mg	

Makes 4 servings

Ingredients:

2 cups black beans, drained, cooked

1 avocado

1 cup cilantro

1 lime, juiced

½ onion, red, chopped

¼ cup sunflower seeds

1 cup cherry tomatoes, halved

Salt

1 tbs olive oil

Directions:

Combine all ingredients in a large bowl. Enjoy.

Nutrition Tip 101: Black beans have a good amount of protein and iron.

ELK TACOS

This recipe may seem a bit eccentric and exotic because of the game meat used, but you may substitute in other types of lean meat. These tacos are very flavorful while being lean.

NUTRITIONAL ANALYSIS PER SERVING:

Calories—432	Carbohydrates—32 g	Vitamin A—7.0 mg	Vitamin E—2.9 IU
Fat—20.4 g	Fiber—8.1 g	Vitamin C—15.4 mg	Folate—153.8 mcg
Sodium—208.8 mg	Sugar—0.8 g	Calcium—59.6 mg	Vitamin B_6—0.9 mg
Potassium—941 mg	Protein—32.2 g	Iron—5.3 mg	Vitamin B_{12}—0.7 mcg
		Vitamin D—0.2 IU	

Makes 1 serving

Ingredients:

3 ounces of elk, strips

1 lime, juiced

½ avocado

2 tbs garlic

1 tsp cumin

½ tsp oregano

½ tsp chili powder

Spelt tortilla

Olive oil

Salt

Directions:

Lay elk on a plate and season with cumin, oregano, and chili powder. Heat a small amount of olive oil in a skillet to medium to high heat. Add garlic and elk. Cook covered for 3 to 5 minutes on each side. Add salt. To the tortilla, add cooked meat, avocado, and a squeeze of lime.

Nutrition Tip 101: Game meat like elk is preferable as an animal protein source because of its higher density of omega 3 fatty acids, its branched chained fatty acids, and its overall lean fat content.

CHANTERELLE AND SHIITAKE SOUP

With its earthy tones, this wild mushroom soup is very satisfying and grounding. It is perfect on days when you desire something light but with texture and minerals to revive your energy.

NUTRITIONAL ANALYSIS PER SERVING:

Calories—213	Sugar—4 g	Vitamin D—0.3 IU
Fat—10.9 g	Protein—5.5 g	Vitamin E—3.4 IU
Sodium—79 mg	Vitamin A—836.5 mg	Folate—72.1 mcg
Potassium—860.3 mg	Vitamin C—51.1 mg	Vitamin B_6—0.3 mg
Carbohydrates—22.4 g	Calcium—104.8 mg	Vitamin B_{12}—0.1 mcg
Fiber—3.4 g	Iron—0.3 mg	

Makes 4 servings

Ingredients:

2 cups chanterelle mushrooms, chopped

2 cups shiitake mushrooms, chopped

1 tbs ghee

4 stalks green onions, chopped

¼ tsp thyme

¼ tsp sage

3 cloves garlic, minced

1 cup parsley, chopped

1 yellow squash, chopped and diced

2 to 4* cups bone or vegetable broth (low sodium)

2 to 3 tbs olive oil

½ cup sherry

Salt to taste

*You can prepare this like a soup or stew depending on how much broth you add. For a more stew-like consistency, pour over a grain or roasted veggies and use less broth.

Directions:

In a pan with 1 TSB olive oil, add the chanterelles, shiitakes, ½ cup of vegetable broth, butter, and sherry. Sauté over medium to high heat until mushrooms become softened. Stir frequently. Remove mixture and place in a bowl. In the same pan, add remaining olive oil, green onions, thyme, sage, parsley, garlic, and squash. Sauté for 5 minutes over medium heat. Add the remaining broth to consistency, along with the mushroom mixture. With all ingredients added, cook for an additional 20 minutes over low to medium heat until the squash has softened. Salt to taste.

Nutrition Tip 101: Wild mushrooms like shiitake have compounds called polysaccharides that help stimulate important parts of the immune system to better fight cancer cells.

STUFFED ACORN SQUASH

Stuffed squash always reminds me of Thanksgiving. You'll be giving thanks for this savory meal that contains a variety of flavors and textures.

NUTRITIONAL ANALYSIS PER SERVING:

Calories—143.6	Sugar—1.6 g	Vitamin D—0 IU
Fat—5 g	Protein—5.6 g	Vitamin E—1.3 IU
Sodium—35.8 mg	Vitamin A—28.6 mg	Folate—46.3 mcg
Potassium—679.4 mg	Vitamin C—18.2 mg	Vitamin B_6—0.3 mg
Carbohydrates—23.6 g	Calcium—70.4 mg	Vitamin B_{12}—0.1 mcg
Fiber—4.1 g	Iron—1.7 mg	

Makes 7 to 8 servings

Ingredients:

2 acorn squash, sliced in half (from end to end, seeds removed)

1 cup wild rice (black rice)

2 cups bone broth

½ cup acorns or filberts

1 onion, chopped

3 stalks celery, chopped

4 cloves garlic, minced

1 tsp sage

1 tsp thyme

Salt

Directions:

Preheat oven to 425°.

Brush squash with olive oil and roast for 35 to 45 minutes. Meanwhile, cook wild rice in bone broth for 45 minutes or until soft. In a skillet, sauté onion, celery, garlic, and acorns or filberts with spices.

When rice is done, add onion mixture. When acorn squash is soft (after 35–45 minutes), remove from heat. Place the rice and onion mixture into the squash cavity. Place back into the oven to bake for 10 to 15 more minutes.

Nutrition Tip 101: Acorn and other squash contain great amounts of soluble fiber, vitamin A, and vitamin C.

SALMON OVER "PASTA"

This dish is a combination of savory fish sauce and "pasta." The zucchini used to make the pasta is sautéed in garlic and basil and then topped by the fragrant fish stewed in coconut milk, cilantro, and lemongrass. It's a delicious meal.

NUTRITIONAL ANALYSIS PER SERVING:

Calories—690	Sugar—12.3 g	Vitamin D—7.7 IU
Fat—56 g	Protein—33.3 g	Vitamin E—3.6 IU
Sodium—131.6 mg	Vitamin A—235.2 mg	Folate—172.7 mcg
Potassium—1858.3 mg	Vitamin C—80.8 mg	Vitamin B_6—1.4 mg
Carbohydrates—19.8 g	Calcium—145 mg	Vitamin B_{12}—3.2 mcg
Fiber—5.9 g	Iron—4.9 mg	

Makes 2 servings

Ingredients:

8 ounces salmon

½ lemon, thinly sliced

½ lime, thinly sliced

16 ounces coconut milk

1 bunch cilantro

2 stalks lemongrass

2 medium to large zucchinis

2 to 3 cloves of garlic, minced

1 cup basil, fresh

Extra virgin olive oil

Directions:

Preheat oven to 400°.

In a blender, mix coconut milk, cilantro, and lemongrass with a pinch of salt. In a medium-sized cast iron skillet or 8x8 inch baking dish, add the fluid. Lay the salmon in the mixture and cook in the oven for about 20 to 30 minutes or until the fish is flakey and cooked.

While the salmon is cooking, shred the zucchini into long thin strips. To a pan, add enough olive oil to sauté the zucchini. Add the garlic and fresh basil to the oil and sauté for 3 minutes. Add the zucchini and cook over medium heat for another 5 minutes. The zucchini should be soft. Add to a plate.

Place the salmon and pan sauce over the zucchini noodles. Enjoy.

Nutrition Tip 101: Cold water fish like salmon contain great levels of omega 3 fatty acids helpful to decrease inflammation and proper immune response.

VEGETABLE POT PIE

This dish is comfort food for the heart and for health. You'll love sinking your teeth into this savory vegetable medley. The textures of the dish vary from crunchy to chewy to smooth. If you like heat with your food, you can add some habanero chili spice to the recipe.

NUTRITIONAL ANALYSIS PER SERVING:

Calories—127	Sugar—2.2 g	Vitamin D—0 IU
Fat—6.3 g	Protein—2.4 g	Vitamin E—0 IU
Sodium—127.4 mg	Vitamin A—230.6 mg	Folate—55.5 mcg
Potassium—204.3 mg	Vitamin C—17.7 mg	Vitamin B_6—0.1 mg
Carbohydrates—16.1 g	Calcium—36.2 mg	Vitamin B_{12}—0 mcg
Fiber—2 g	Iron—1.2 mg	

Makes 6 servings

Ingredients:

2 rice flour pie crusts

2 cups spinach, chopped

1 cup broccoli, chopped

1 cup carrots

2 cups sweet potatoes, cubed, roasted

1 cup shiitake mushrooms, chopped

3 cloves garlic, minced

1 tbs sage

Gravy over grain recipe (page 49)

Optional: habanero, dried spice

Directions:

Preheat oven to 425°.

Make the Gravy Over Grain recipe found on page 49. Mix vegetables and mushrooms in a large bowl. Once the gravy cooks for approximately 20 minutes, add the vegetables and cook for another 20 minutes or until vegetables are slightly soft. Add sage and garlic. At this point, you can add the desired amount of habanero to the vegetables. If too soupy, you can drain some of the liquid off. Pour vegetable mixture over one pie crust in a pie plate. Cover the vegetables with the second pie crust. Bake for 25 to 30 minutes. Let sit for 10 to 15 minutes before serving.

Nutrition Tip 101: Spinach is a good source of not only iron but also of calcium and magnesium.

SMOTHERED LIVER

Either you love it, hate it, or have never tried it. For people who like liver, this is a great recipe that is simplistic yet healthful, especially when eaten in moderation. The strong liver flavor is mellowed by being first soaked in whole milk and then being smothered by sweet white onions.

NUTRITIONAL ANALYSIS PER SERVING:

Calories—254.4	Carbohydrates—6.2 g	Vitamin A—421.4 mg	Vitamin E—1.6 IU
Fat—27.3 g	Fiber—0.2 g	Vitamin C—0.9 mg	Folate—51.7 mcg
Sodium—296.6 mg	Sugar—0 g	Calcium—31 mg	Vitamin B_6—0 mg
Potassium—66.5 mg	Protein—7.0 g	Iron—2.8 mg	Vitamin B_{12}—1.7 mcg
		Vitamin D—0.3 IU	

Makes 4 servings

Ingredients:

3 to 4 livers, beef, organic, grass-fed   Olive oil

Whole milk, enough to cover liver   ½ tsp paprika

1 cup spelt flour   Black pepper

1 white onion, sliced   Salt

Directions:

Soak liver in whole milk for 20 to 30 minutes.

While the liver is soaking, sauté the onions in a pan with olive oil until they are translucent. Remove from heat and place in a covered bowl.

Remove the liver from the milk and season with paprika, salt, and pepper on both sides. To a tray, add the flour. Coat both sides of the liver in flour. In a pan, heat enough olive oil enough to fry over medium to high heat. Add the liver and cook for 3 to 4 minutes per side. The liver should be neither too tough nor too juicy.

Nutritional Tip 101: Liver is an excellent source of iron and B_{12}. It is very important to use organic free-range beef.

MUSSELS WITH WHITE WINE AND THYME

There is an ease involved in making this dish that does not match its delicious flavor. The meal mixes earthy notes of fresh herbs and wine blended to perfection. The resulting broth, infused with fresh thyme and parsley, are great for dipping a hearty homemade sourdough bread.

NUTRITIONAL ANALYSIS PER SERVING:

Calories—241	Protein—27.9 g	Magnesium—88 mg
Fat—9 g	Iron—9.73 mg	Potassium—832 mg
Carbohydrates—10.5 g	Sodium—688 mg	Vitamin C—25.9 mg
Fiber—1.2 g	Calcium—83 mg	Folate—106 mcg

Makes 4 servings

Ingredients:

2 pounds of mussels

2 tbs ghee or butter

¼ cup minced scallions

1 tbs thyme

1 tbs minced garlic

¼ cup of parsley

1 cup of white wine

Directions:

Clean mussels by scrubbing with a brush under cool water. Discard any that are opened. Set aside.

In a skillet, sauté scallions, garlic, and ghee for 5 minutes or until slightly browned. Add 1 cup of white wine and allow to simmer for 5 to 10 minutes. Add mussels, cover skillet, and cook until mussels open. Stir in fresh thyme and parsley. Enjoy.

Nutrition Tip 101: This recipe contains an excellent amount of omega 3 fatty acids, branched chained amino acids, selenium, manganese, and vitamins K and B$_{12}$.

SAUERKRAUT SOUP

Thanks to several patients with Slavic backgrounds, I was turned on to this fantastic soup-stew. It is hearty and warming. The overall preparation process mellows out the tanginess of the sauerkraut. If you like sauerkraut, you'll love this recipe.

NUTRITIONAL ANALYSIS PER SERVING:

Calories—96.1	Sugar—5.4 g	Vitamin D—0 IU
Fat—13.3 g	Protein—5.1 g	Vitamin E—0.4 IU
Sodium—604 mg	Vitamin A—477.8 mg	Folate—32.2 mcg
Potassium—518.2 mg	Vitamin C—15.6 mg	Vitamin B_6—0.2 mg
Carbohydrates—18.3 g	Calcium—55.3 mg	Vitamin B_{12}—0.2 mcg
Fiber—4.5 g	Iron—1.9 mg	

Makes 6 servings

Ingredients:

1 medium onion, diced

2 bay leaves

2 medium carrots, peeled and sliced

2 medium sweet potatoes, peeled and diced

4 cups base bone broth (page 62) or store-bought broth

2 cups water

2 cups sauerkraut

Optional: Chicken sausage

Salt and pepper, to taste

Directions:

To a large pot over medium-high heat, add the onion and about a ¼ to ½ cup of the bone broth. Sauté until the onions are soft. Add the bay leaves and stir. Add the carrots, sweet potatoes, remaining bone broth, water, and sauerkraut and bring to a boil. Reduce the heat to medium-low and partially cover. Simmer until the sweet potatoes and carrots are tender, which will be about 15 to 20 minutes. Taste and add salt and pepper.

BLACK BEAN BURGER

Look no farther for a fantastic tasting vegetarian burger. This burger is fun to make and also to eat. It contains a variety of spices that'll make you forget that you are eating beans.

NUTRITIONAL ANALYSIS PER SERVING:

Calories—219	Sugar—1.7 g	Vitamin D—0.3 IU
Fat—13.3 g	Protein—7.7 g	Vitamin E—2.4 IU
Sodium—315 mg	Vitamin A—64.2 mg	Folate—93.6 mcg
Potassium—297.0 mg	Vitamin C—5.2 mg	Vitamin B_6—0.1 mg
Carbohydrates—18.7 g	Calcium—38.7 mg	Vitamin B_{12}—0.3 mcg
Fiber—4.3 g	Iron—1.6 mg	

Makes 4 to 5 servings

Ingredients:

16 ounces black beans	2 eggs
¼ to ½ cup extra virgin olive oil	½ cup cilantro
1 cup red onions, chopped	1 tsp cumin
4 cloves garlic, minced	½ cup wild rice
1 tsp chili powder	Salt

Directions:

Preheat oven to 325°.

Spread beans on a cookie sheet and roast them for about 15 minutes to dry them out a bit. While the beans are in the oven, sauté onions and garlic in 1 to 2 tbs of olive oil. Remove beans and increase the oven temperature to 375° for later.

To a blender or food processor, add the beans, onion and garlic mixture, and all the other ingredients. If you need more moisture, add additional olive oil. Using about 1/3 of a cup of the mixture, form into patties. Place on cookie platter.

Bake at 375° for 10 minutes each side.

Nutrition Tip 101: Eggs contain a good amount of protein and also folate. Both are needed in the production of red blood cells.

SIDES

GRAVY OVER GRAIN

This gravy is light with a slightly cheesy flavor. Unlike conventional gravies, this one does not contain a great deal of oil. The essential oils from sage, garlic, and turmeric combine perfectly to make a great cover over rice or quinoa.

NUTRITIONAL ANALYSIS PER SERVING:

Calories—158.7	Sugar—1.0 g	Vitamin D—0 IU
Fat—8.3 g	Protein—3.8 g	Vitamin E—1.4 IU
Sodium—5.2 mg	Vitamin A—0.1 mg	Folate—35.9 mcg
Potassium—114.4 mg	Vitamin C—0.8 mg	Vitamin B_6—2.0 mg
Carbohydrates—18.1 g	Calcium—8.4 mg	Vitamin B_{12}—1.2 mcg
Fiber—1.7 g	Iron—0.7 mg	

Makes 6 to 8 servings

Ingredients:

⅓ cup chickpea flour

⅓ cup nutritional yeast flakes

¼ cup extra virgin olive oil

2 cups vegetable broth

Sage

Garlic, minced

Turmeric, powder

Salt to taste

3 cups quinoa or wild rice, cooked

Directions:

Add olive oil to a pan and turn heat to medium to high. Add garlic and sauté for about 5 minutes. Add flour, yeast flakes, turmeric, and sage and brown for another 3 to 4 minutes. Decrease heat to simmer. Add vegetable broth and mix. Let ingredients simmer for 20 minutes, stirring frequently. Serve over quinoa or wild rice.

Nutrition Tip 101: Nutritional yeast is brewer's yeast supplemented with many B vitamins.

ROASTED GREEN BEANS

Roasting green beans causes them to slightly caramelize and adds some crunch and chewiness. The spices used in this recipe add savory flavor with a little heat.

NUTRITIONAL ANALYSIS PER SERVING:

Calories—142	Sugar—3.8 g	Vitamin D—0 IU
Fat—10.8 g	Protein—3.6 g	Vitamin E—0.6 IU
Sodium—10.3 mg	Vitamin A—53.9 mg	Folate—48.9 mcg
Potassium—293.6 mg	Vitamin C—14.9 mg	Vitamin B_6—0.2 mg
Carbohydrates—10.4 g	Calcium—62.1 mg	Vitamin B_{12}—0 mcg
Fiber—4.5 g	Iron—2.0 mg	

Makes 4 servings

Ingredients:

1 pound green beans, frozen or fresh, cut into half or fourths

2 tbs sesame seed oil

½ cup basil

¼ cup sesame seeds

1 tbs ginger, fresh, shredded

2 tbs chili flakes

Directions:

Preheat oven to 375°.

In a bowl combine oil, sesame seeds, ginger, and chili flakes. Mix. Add green beans and coat beans with mixture. Spread green beans onto a baking sheet and place in the oven. Roast for 30 to 40 minutes. Remove from heat and transfer to a bowl. Mix in basil, which will wilt from heat of the green beans. Enjoy.

Nutrition Tip 101: Basil contains essential oils like eugenol that is anti-inflammatory.

ROASTED KOHLRABI

You've all seen this vegetable in your grocery stores and probably wondered what in the world would I do with that. Here you have a recipe for the delicious kohlrabi, or German turnip. It belongs to the cruciferous vegetable family and as a result tastes like a cross between cabbage and broccoli. When roasted, the vegetable caramelizes, mellows, and sweetens.

NUTRITIONAL ANALYSIS PER SERVING:

Calories—158.2	Carbohydrates—8.7 g	Vitamin A—2.8 mg	Vitamin E—2.7 IU
Fat—13.7 g	Fiber—5 g	Vitamin C—86.8 mg	Folate—22.4 mcg
Sodium—28.3 mg	Sugar—3.6 g	Calcium—33.7 mg	Vitamin B_6—0.2 mg
Potassium—490.1 mg	Protein—2.4 g	Iron—0.6 mg	Vitamin B_{12}—0 mcg
		Vitamin D—0 IU	

Makes 2 servings

Ingredients:

Kohlrabi	Salt
2 tbs olive oil	Pepper

Directions:

Heat oven to 375°.

Slice Kohlrabi and place in a bowl. Add olive oil, salt and pepper, and toss. Cook for 15 to 20 minutes. Enjoy.

Nutrition Tip 101: Kohlrabi is in the same family as cabbage and broccoli and thus contains some of the important and helpful estrogen regulating compounds.

TAHINI AND COLLARD GREENS

This recipe is another one of my favorite because of its ease of preparation, and its taste. Collard greens can have a sharp, rich taste. Adding tahini and lemon mellow this flavor out to perfection. This dish is an excellent source of calcium.

NUTRITIONAL ANALYSIS PER SERVING:

Calories—456.6	Sugar—3.8 g	Vitamin D—0 IU
Fat—35.1 g	Protein—15.6 g	Vitamin E—2.2 IU
Sodium—129.1 mg	Vitamin A—1035.5 mg	Folate—103.7 mcg
Potassium—901/3 mg	Vitamin C—169.7 mg	Vitamin B_6—0.5 mg
Carbohydrates—24.9 g	Calcium—450.7 mg	Vitamin B_{12}—0 mcg
Fiber—9.7 g	Iron—8.0 mg	

Makes 2 servings

Ingredients:

1 bunch collard greens, thinly sliced

1 lemon, squeezed, juice

½ cup tahini

1 tbs garlic, minced

1 tbs sesame seeds

½ tsp chili flakes

Salt

Directions:

To the collard greens, add ½ tsp of salt. Massage the salt into the greens and let them sit for about 5 to 10 minutes. Next, add lemon juice and mix well. Then add the tahini, garlic, sesame seeds, and chili flakes. Mix. Let the entire mixture sit for 20 more minutes, covered at room temperature. Enjoy.

Nutrition Tip 101: Besides being an excellent source of fiber, collard greens are also a great source of calcium. More calcium can be released and made more available by adding vinegar to the vegetable before eating or during cooking.

STUFFED SWEET POTATO

Reminiscent of a baked potato with "everything," this healthful recipe will leave you satisfied in the best way. The taste combination is very different from the standard potato, however, with more of a Middle Eastern or Mediterranean flare. The high protein content is a plus.

NUTRITIONAL ANALYSIS PER SERVING:

Calories—434.4	Sugar—14.5 g	Vitamin D—0 IU
Fat—17.9 g	Protein—13.9 g	Vitamin E—1.6 IU
Sodium—103.4 mg	Vitamin A—1745.2 mg	Folate—141.3 mcg
Potassium—1159.7 mg	Vitamin C—37 mg	Vitamin B_6—0.6 mg
Carbohydrates—59.3 g	Calcium—233.2 mg	Vitamin B_{12}—0 mcg
Fiber—11.4 g	Iron—5.7 mg	

Makes 4 servings

Ingredients:

4 sweet potatoes, medium

16 ounces chick peas

2 tbs garlic, minced

½ cup basil, fresh

1 tsp turmeric, dry spice

½ cup tahini

Salt

Squeeze of lemon juice

Optional: brush with sesame seed oil

Directions:

Preheat oven to 375°.

Steam 2 medium-size sweet potatoes until soft. Scoop out the center of the potato, leaving approximately a half inch of flesh on the skin.

To a blender, add the sweet potato that you have scooped out, chick peas, garlic, tahini, turmeric, and basil. Blend until pureed. Salt to taste.

Place the puree back into the potato skins. At this point, you can choose to brush the mixture with some sesame seed oil or drizzle it on.

Bake for 20 minutes. Remove from oven and add a squeeze of lemon before serving. Enjoy.

Nutrition Tip 101: Chick peas, also known as garbanzo beans, contain an excellent amount of protein and are extremely versatile in plant-based cooking. They can be used as a bean or ground to be used as a flour in baking.

CREAMED CARROTS, PARSNIPS, AND GINGER

This pleasant side dish is a smooth and spicy take on mashed potatoes. Parsnips have a sweet, nutty flavor, while carrots are sweet. The addition of ginger adds some heat to the earthy taste of this recipe.

NUTRITIONAL ANALYSIS PER SERVING:

Calories—137.6	Sugar—6.3 g	Vitamin D—0 IU
Fat—7.1 g	Protein—1.4 g	Vitamin E—1.5 IU
Sodium—51.2 mg	Vitamin A—534.4 mg	Folate—57 mcg
Potassium—466.6 mg	Vitamin C—15.2 mg	Vitamin B_6—0.2 mg
Carbohydrates—18.6 g	Calcium—45.5 mg	Vitamin B_{12}—0 mcg
Fiber—3.9 g	Iron—0.6 mg	

Makes 4 servings

Ingredients:

2 cups carrots, uncooked, chopped

2 cups parsnips, uncooked, chopped

2 tbs ginger, shredded

2 tbs sesame seed oil

Salt to taste

Directions:

Steam carrots and parsnips until soft. Place steamed vegetables, ginger, and oil into a blender or food processor and mix until even consistency. Add salt to taste. Serve warm.

Nutrition Tip 101: Carrots have a great amount to vitamin A and beta-carotene which are helpful for tissue healing and also eyesight.

PLUM CHUTNEY

You may want to include this succulent condiment as a staple with your lunch and dinner meals. It is sweet and tangy and serves to bring out the flavors of your favorite foods. This delightful dish contains good levels of vitamin C, iron, and potassium. It is also a good source of soluble fiber.

NUTRITIONAL ANALYSIS PER SERVING:

Calories—83	Protein—0.8 g	Magnesium—8 mg
Fat—0.3 g	Iron—0.3 mg	Potassium—144 mg
Carbohydrates—20.9 g	Sodium—147 mg	Vitamin C—7.6 mg
Fiber—1.3 g	Calcium—11 mg	Folate—7 mcg

Makes 8 servings

Ingredients:

8 plums, sliced and halved, skin on, discard pit

1 medium red onion, coarsely chopped

⅓ cup dried currants

¼ cup apple cider vinegar

2 large garlics, cut paper thin

1 tsp mustard seed

½ tsp salt

½ tsp ground black pepper

½ cup water

⅓ cup honey

Directions:

Bring ½ cup of water to a boil. Place plums into pot with boiling water. When it boils again, add all other ingredients. Cook for 25 to 30 minutes until most of the liquid has been cooked off of the mixture.

Nutritional Tip 101: Plums contain the healthy compounds sorbitol and isatin. Known health benefits include regulating the functioning of the digestive system. Plums are also a source of vitamin A, beta-carotene, and phenolic antioxidants (zeaxanthin) which are essential in eyesight and in the prevention of lung and oral cavity cancers.

DESSERTS

CHERRY AND CHOCOLATE BARS

Every once in a while we want something fancy, a little cheat. This recipe does contain a greater amount of sugar, but it also contains a decent amount of protein and good fats to keep the insulin surge at a bump rather than a peak.

NUTRITIONAL ANALYSIS PER SERVING:

Calories—395.6	Sugar—17 g	Vitamin D—0 IU
Fat—25.5 g	Protein—8.1 g	Vitamin E—0.5 IU
Sodium—23.0 mg	Vitamin A—9.0 mg	Folate—138.7 mcg
Potassium—345.8 mg	Vitamin C—0.8 mg	Vitamin B_6—0.2 mg
Carbohydrates—37.5 g	Calcium—43.4 mg	Vitamin B_{12}—0 mcg
Fiber—5.9 g	Iron—2.3 mg	

Makes 6 servings

Ingredients:

16 ounces cherries (in water), Montmorency or tart, drained

½ cup dark chocolate chips, unsweetened

½ cup coconut oil

2 cups almond (blanched) flour

2 tbs chia seeds

3 tbs coconut sugar

1 pinch of salt

Directions:

Preheat oven to 350°.

In a bowl, combine almond flour, chia seeds, coconut sugar, salt, and coconut oil. Mix. It might be helpful to melt the coconut oil before mixing. Increase or decrease the amount of almond flour to make the crust to stick together.

Press half of the crust mixture into the greased pan. Layer the drained cherries and the chocolate over the crust. Crumble the remaining crust mixture on top of the cherries and chocolate until covered. Press the mixture gently to form an even crust.

Place in oven and cook for 30 to 40 minutes. The top should be golden brown. Take pan from oven and cool for 20 minutes. Enjoy.

Nutrient Tip 101: Chia seeds are a fantastic and versatile food, especially in plant-based diets. They contain a good amount of protein and soluble fiber that can be added to many recipes.

CHERRY CRUMBLE

This simple dessert is easy to make. The fancy recipe is all about the cherries!

NUTRITIONAL ANALYSIS PER SERVING:

Calories—86.3	Carbohydrates—9.9 g	Vitamin A—6.4 mg	Vitamin E—0.2 IU
Fat—4.8 g	Fiber—1.2 g	Vitamin C—0.5 mg	Folate—28 mcg
Sodium—4.9 mg	Sugar—4.1 g	Calcium—6.6 mg	Vitamin B_6—0 mg
Potassium—101.1 mg	Protein—1.8 g	Iron—0.5 mg	Vitamin B_{12}—0 mcg
		Vitamin D—0 IU	

Makes 6 to 8 servings

Ingredients:

Filling
10 ounces frozen or canned cherries
1 tbs date sugar
1 tbs tapioca flour
Crust

½ cup almond flour
½ cup coconut, shredded
2 tbs dates, dried
2 tbs coconut oil
2 tbs cashews

Directions:

Preheat oven to 350°.

Combine and mix crust ingredients in a blender. The mixture should stick together enough to be pressed into a ball. If not, add more coconut oil. When the correct consistency is achieved, press crust dough into the bottom of the oven pan.

In a separate bowl, combine the filling ingredients. Mix well and spread on crust. Bake in oven for 35 to 40 minutes or until the fruit is bubbling. Cool for 20 minutes.

Nutrient Tip 101: Cherries contain a good number of phytonutrients, some of which are anti-inflammatories and other assist in lowering pain.

BAKED BANANAS WITH CINNAMON AND CHOCOLATE

Every once in a while we'd like to have a dessert. This recipe provides sweet taste while helping to control blood sugar. But don't be fooled, this dish is decadent with its dark chocolate and aromatic spices of cardamom and cinnamon. A little goes a long way.

NUTRITIONAL ANALYSIS PER SERVING:

Calories—195	Fiber—2.8 g	Sodium—14 mg	Potassium—281 mg
Total Fat—7.3 g	Protein—1.3 g	Calcium—15 mg	Vitamin C—6.3 mg
Carbohydrates—34 g	Iron—0.7 mg	Magnesium—33 mg	Vitamin D—0 IU
			Folate—9 mcg

Makes 4 servings

Ingredients:

2 bananas, sliced into halves

1 tsp cardamom

1 tsp cinnamon

2 tbs coconut oil

¼ cup chocolate, dark

Directions:

Heat oven to 375°.

Place banana slices on a cookie sheet. Add the coconut oil, cardamom, and cinnamon to the bananas. Bake for 15 minutes. While the bananas are baking, melt chocolate. Drizzle the chocolate onto the bananas when they come out of the oven. Enjoy.

Nutrition Tip 101: Dark chocolate contains anti-inflammatory polyphenols and a number of other beneficial nutrients, including magnesium. Organic chocolate is the best.

SNACKS

BROCCOLI AND CHICKPEAS WITH TAHINI DIP

This delicious dip is a twist on hummus which makes it a little more interesting. By adding broccoli, the nutrient content increases and the vegetable adds some fun texture too.

NUTRITIONAL ANALYSIS PER SERVING:

Calories—250.1	Sugar—1.6 g	Vitamin D—0 IU
Fat—20.6 g	Protein—6.2 g	Vitamin E—1.6 IU
Sodium—29.2 mg	Vitamin A—13.7 mg	Folate—74.9 mcg
Potassium—207 mg	Vitamin C—10.8 mg	Vitamin B_6—0.1 mg
Carbohydrates—13.0 g	Calcium—109 mg	Vitamin B_{12}—0 mcg
Fiber—3.4 g	Iron—2.9 mg	

Makes 6 servings

Ingredients:

1 cup chickpeas, cooked or canned
½ cup tahini
¼ cup olive oil or avocado oil
4 garlic cloves, large, minced

1 lemon, juiced
½ cup broccoli, florets, chopped
¼ cup parsley
Optional: ⅛ tsp habanero chili, dried spice

Directions:

In a pan, at medium to high heat, add olive oil, sauté broccoli and garlic until slightly soft. Add broccoli and garlic to a blender, and then add all other ingredients and blend.

Nutrient Tip 101: Broccoli is high in vitamin C and also calcium.

STUFFED AVOCADOS

How great are avocados, you might ask? They are almost perfect. In this recipe, they live up to the rating. This dish is easy to make, buttery, and satisfyingly good.

NUTRITIONAL ANALYSIS PER SERVING:

Calories 501	Protein—45.72 g	Potassium—1259 mg
Total Fat—25.7 g	Iron—1.95 mg	Vitamin C—13 mg
Carbohydrates—11.5 g	Sodium—944 mg	Folate—92 mcg
Fiber—7.4 g	Calcium—446 mg	

Makes 2 servings

Ingredients:

1 avocado

6 ounces salmon, cooked

½ cup cilantro, chopped

2 cloves garlic, minced

¼ onion, finely chopped

½ lemon, juice from

1 tsp aioli

1 celery stalk, chopped

Directions:

Put salmon in a bowl. Add garlic, onions, aioli, celery, cilantro, and lemon juice. Mix. Slice an avocado in half. Remove the seed. Fill each avocado half with salmon mixture. Enjoy.

Nutrition Tip 101: This recipe contains a good amount of tryptophan and other branched chain amino acids; vitamins B_3, B_6, B_{12}, and D; and selenium.

BLACK-EYED PEA DIP

This dip is similar to hummus but is made with black beans for variety. The texture is a little more substantial, but the flavor is still delicious. This is a quick and easy recipe to make—two steps: blend and serve!

NUTRITIONAL ANALYSIS PER SERVING:

Calories—43	Carbohydrates—8 g	Vitamin A—21.4 mg	Vitamin E—0.1 IU
Fat—0.3 g	Fiber—1.4 g	Vitamin C—10.4 mg	Folate—51.0 mcg
Sodium—9.0 mg	Sugar—0.7 g	Calcium—19.5 mg	Vitamin B_6—0.1 mg
Potassium—163.0 mg	Protein—8.1 g	Iron—1.2 mg	Vitamin B_{12}—0 mcg
		Vitamin D—0 IU	

Makes 6 servings

Ingredients:

1 cup black-eyed peas, cooked

½ cup parsley, chopped

2 garlic cloves

½ cup onions

¼ cup tahini

2 tbs lemon juice

Salt to taste

Directions:

Put all ingredients into a blender. Mix until consistency is even. Add water if the mixture begins to clump.

Nutrition Tip 101: Black-eyed peas are an excellent source of calcium, potassium, and fiber. The soluble fiber in black-eyed peas are helpful in cholesterol control.

BASE BROTH

If you are my patient, you'd be on broth daily at some point in your treatment protocol. Broth contains an excellent dose of electrolytes and minerals. A daily cup is refreshing and rejuvenating.

NUTRITIONAL ANALYSIS PER SERVING:

Calories—16.8	Carbohydrates—0 g	Vitamin A—500 mg	Vitamin E—0 IU
Fat—0 g	Fiber—0 g	Vitamin C—1.0 mg	Folate—7.2 mcg
Sodium—554.4 mg	Sugar—0.5 g	Calcium—19.2 mg	Vitamin B_6—0 mg
Potassium—204 mg	Protein—3.3 g	Iron—0.6 mg	Vitamin B_{12}—0 mcg
		Vitamin D—0 IU	

Makes 6 servings

Ingredients:

1 cup chopped okra

1 bunch parsley, chopped

1 bunch cilantro, chopped

1 bunch beet greens (from about 4 beets), chopped

4 carrots

1 onion

1 garlic

2 tbs of blackstrap molasses, organic

8 quarts of water

Chicken (or turkey) bones (at least six up to whole carcass)

Directions:

To a large pot, add water, bones, vegetables, and molasses. Simmer for 8 to 12 hours (or longer). If water decreases more than 1/3 the level of the starting volume, add amount that evaporated. Broth keeps in the refrigerator for about 5 days and in the freezer for about 3 months.

Nutrient Tip 101: Blackstrap molasses contains a good source of elemental minerals such as iron, calcium, potassium, and magnesium. A daily cup is restorative for everyone.

REJUVENATION JUICE

*I love this green drink. Besides being refreshing, it is packed with minerals and acts
as a mild diuretic. It has an earthy taste and is brightened with lemon and pear juice.*

Makes 1 serving

Ingredients:

½ bunch parsley
½ bunch cilantro
3 stalks celery

½ bunch dandelion leaves (seasonal;
if available)
½ lemon
½ pear

Directions:

Juice all ingredients in a juicer. Mix well. Enjoy.

I would recommend not to have this drink at night, as it is a slight diuretic and
may interrupt your sleep because of added bathroom calls.

Nutrition Tip 101: Dandelion leaves and the juice from leaves are diuretic yet contain
a great source of potassium. In addition, dandelion is bitter, thus helping with proper
and optimal digestion.

Basil-ed Eggs and Yams, p. 28

Breakfast in a Jar, p. 29

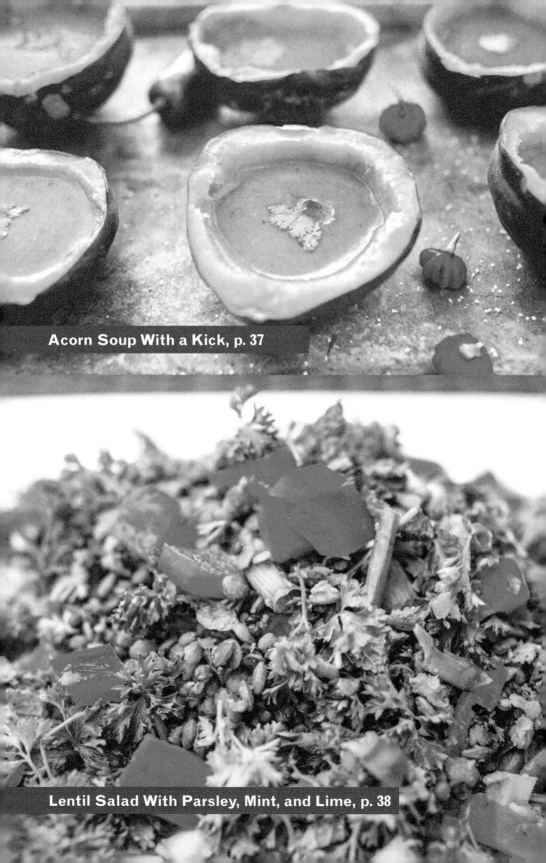

Acorn Soup With a Kick, p. 37

Lentil Salad With Parsley, Mint, and Lime, p. 38

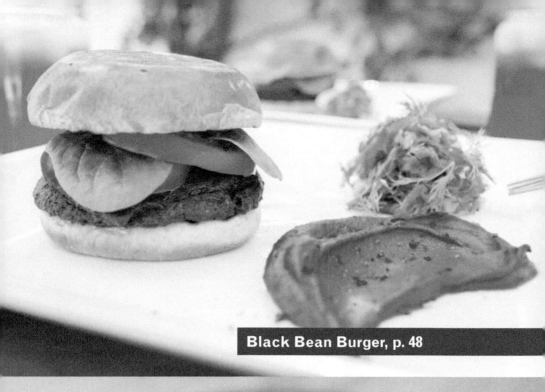

Black Bean Burger, p. 48

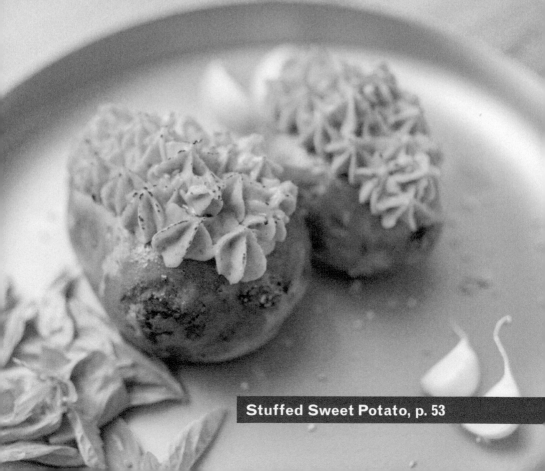

Stuffed Sweet Potato, p. 53

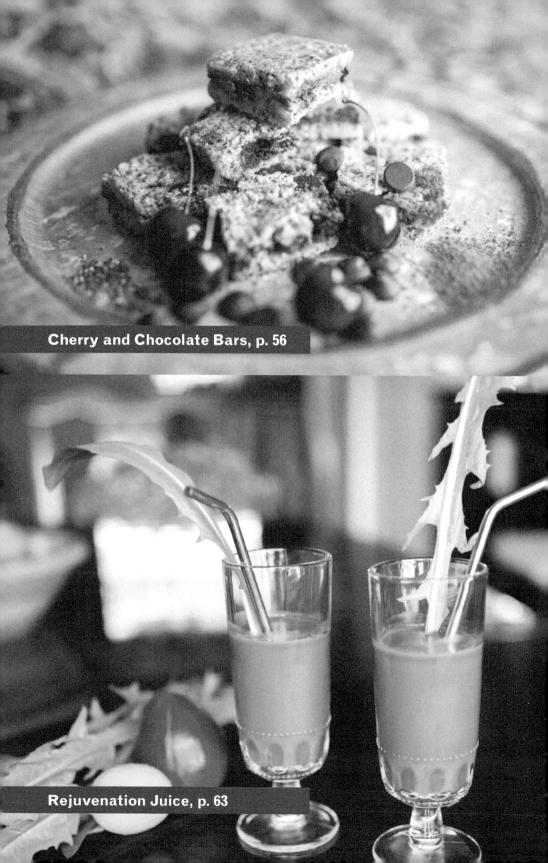

Cherry and Chocolate Bars, p. 56

Rejuvenation Juice, p. 63

CHAPTER 4

Getting Stronger: Exercise for Patients With Breast Cancer

Because if you take a risk, you just might find what you're looking for.

—Susane Colasanti

A well-rounded exercise plan that includes physical activity at least 5 days a week delivers solid health benefits for breast cancer patients and survivors. Physical activity decreases inflammation, boosts the immune system, and stimulates loss in body fat. All these are associated with a decrease in breast cancer risk.

Exercise has been shown to affect treatment outcome and overall quality of life for patients. Studies show that there is an inverse relationship between exercise and the development, or recurrence, of cancer. There are multiple reasons for good treatment outcomes, side effect prevention and reduction for breast cancer patients, and improved quality of life.

Exercise enhances physical function and can slow and stop bone mass loss. Improved physical function is particularly important for patients who have been diagnosed with hormone-sensitive cancers and who are placed on hormone-blocking therapies, and especially for younger cancer patients. Bone loss and osteoporosis are common long-term side effects of treatment. However, studies have shown that weight-bearing exercise, including resistance training, can slow or prevent bone loss. Exercise that targets the upper body can improve range of motion that may have been affected by surgery or radiation. Exercise initiated early after surgery is associated with a decrease in the development of lymphedema.

Patients using chemotherapies that are cardiotoxic, like Adriamycin, can decrease the effects using aerobic exercise. Other side effects, such as nausea, pain, fatigue, and depression, can be reduced with an exercise regimen. Exercise causes the release of endorphins, enkephalins, and serotonin. These hormones act to reduce pain and increase the sensation of feeling good.

In addition, other anti-inflammatory proteins are released that help the immune system in its fight against cancer.

Some patients on hormone therapy will develop joint pain. Exercise helps to reduce or prevent this symptom.

Exercise results in a reduction in estrogen and progesterone and a reduction in adipose (fat) cells. Adipose tissue manufactures and secretes estrogen. That is why having a higher amount of muscle to fat is better for cancer patients and is associated with a decreased risk of occurrence. Exercise also helps to regulate the body's level of insulin secretion and other hormones linked to cancer growth and aggressiveness.

In summary, exercise is extremely important for breast cancer patients and survivors. I believe it should be a prescription.

Let us take a look at some of the most beneficial exercises for breast cancer patients.

WALKING

Brisk walking is a great exercise for breast cancer patients and for increasing the chances of remission. It is aerobic, weight bearing, free, and requires little special equipment.

According to the American Cancer Society, studies link walking to a lower risk of developing breast cancer. Specifically, what studies have found is that at least 7 hours per week of walking is associated with a 14% lowered risk of developing breast cancer after menopause for both overweight and normal range women. A moderate pace of about 3 miles per hour for 25 to 30 minutes a day is enough to see improvements. Adding a faster, brisker pace will actually increase the benefit by up to 25%, according to these studies.

Walking, as well as other exercise, has to be consistent to reap the benefits. A study from Harvard Health Publishing, which was conducted over 17 years, found that if patients stopped exercising the risk-reducing benefits disappeared.

Summary of benefits of walking

- Weight bearing to help strengthen bones (osteopenia and osteoporosis prevention)
- Aerobic, thus increasing circulation and regulating weight
- Improves balance
- Strengthens muscles and improves stamina

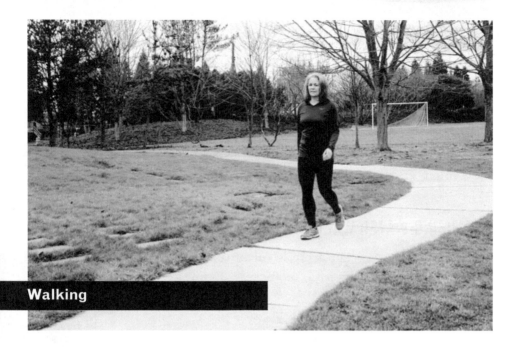

Walking

- Decreases the risk of developing blood clots
- Improves mood and self-esteem
- Decreases nausea

Before starting a walking plan, be sure that you are cleared from your healthcare provider. Make sure you have proper walking gear: comfortable shoes, or sturdy sneakers, and comfortable clothing. Before starting, especially if you are a beginner or have been inactive for a period of time, start by doing lower body stretches for at least 15 minutes. You will want to eventually get to 50% to 60% of maximum heart rate capacity. A personal trainer or your local gym staff should be able to assist you further with proper stretching and your target heart rate.

Most importantly, do not overdo it. We do not want to take two steps forward and five backward.

Brisk Walking Plan

Beginners: Walk for a total of 10 to 15 minutes five times a week. Find a relatively flat place to walk for weeks 1 to 2. After week 2, increase your total walking minutes to 20 minutes and add a hill or two to your walk.

Intermediate: Walk for a total of 20 minutes on a route with at least two hills. Vary the route after week 2 and add another 5 to 10 minutes to the total time of your walk. You should be at about 50% to 60% of maximum heart rate for about 15 to 20 minutes of your total walking time.

Advanced: Walk for a total of 30 to 40 minutes on a route with at least two hills at 50% to 60% of maximum heart rate. After week 2, increase your walking time by 10 more minutes. You can add carrying a backpack with a couple of water bottles in it to increase weight bearing for osteoporosis prevention.

SWIMMING/WATER WALKING

Swimming is an excellent exercise for breast cancer patients, particularly those who have joint injuries, or those who are looking for a total body workout.

Summary of benefits of swimming

- Improves heart health (especially important for patients taking Herceptin and/or Adriamycin)
- Decreases blood pressure

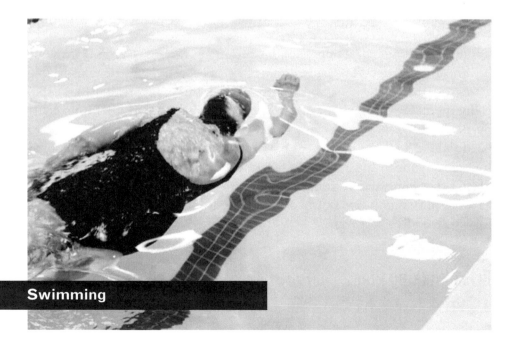

Swimming

- Improves lung capacity
- Increases muscle strength and tone
- Increases bone strength

Swimming helps with weight control and improves high density lipoproteins (HDL) the good cholesterol and decreases low density lipoproteins (LDL) the cholesterol that can cause some problems with heart disease. During swimming, you are working out multiple muscle groups and thus providing cardio and strength training. Swimming helps fight against depression and thus can help with the effects of hormone therapy. Because it is gentle, swimming after breast surgery is an excellent way to exercise all your muscle groups and avoid muscular atrophy, which is quite common during treatment.

Swimming plan postsurgery:

Start slow, especially if you are a beginner. Your workout should include a warm-up and cool down consisting of slower strokes and heart rate and some stretching. Your goal should be 20 to 30 minutes.

Water Walking

Another way to work out in the water is by water walking. It is just like it sounds—walking in water. During lap swimming, secure a lane for yourself. You may want to wear water footies for a better grip on the floor of the pool and a floatation device around your waist.

Beginners: Begin with doing four to five laps (up and back) in the pool. Do not worry about how fast you are going. You want to get used to the water and walking.

Intermediate: Your goal is now 20 minutes with a maximum heart rate of 50% to 60%.

Advanced: Your goal is 30 to 40 minutes with a maximum heart rate of 50% to 60%.

RESISTANCE TRAINING

Resistance training is any exercise that causes the muscles to contract against an external resistance with the expectation of increases in strength, tone, mass, and/or endurance. Resistance training makes your muscles work harder by adding weight or resistance.

Resistance training is great for postcancer adverse side effects. One of the side effects of breast cancer treatment is an accelerated bone mineral density. This symptom is associated with hormone therapy treatment and chemically (chemotherapy) induced menopause. Resistance training has been shown to be a safe and effective way to slow bone loss and prevent osteoporosis, and may serve as an effective alternative to pharmaceutical treatment. Studies have found that bone density levels were well maintained with training. Resistance training can also help fix muscle imbalances or weakness after breast cancer treatment.

A study showed resistance training results in improved physical function and quality of life in breast cancer patients. Patients with breast cancer or metastatic disease participated in a study by conducting a 60-minute strength training session and aerobic exercise twice a week. Researchers found that participants reduced pain and fatigue at the 3- and 6-month marks.

Resistance training has been shown to be safe for breast cancer survivors with no increase of lymphedema.

There are various types of resistance training one can choose from. Following are some examples and an example beginning plan.

Free weight lifting. These exercises use handheld weights which are lifted in various positions to target specific muscles. The exercises are usually done in repetition until the muscle is more or less fatigued. This exercise can be done in the gym or at home. You can lift manufactured hand weights or anything weighted, like cans of food or gallon jugs of water.

Weight machines. Resistance training using weight machines requires special equipment which can be found in public or private gyms. Weight machines require some basic training to execute the exercises safely and effectively. You can hire a trainer or ask for assistance from the on-staff attendant at the gym. Like free weights, lifts are done in repetition until the muscles are more or less fatigued.

Suggested Beginning Resistant Exercise Plan

Resistance exercise will depend on your level of fitness and range of motion. Your end goal should be about 30 to 40 minutes four times a week. I recommend that you start out with a trainer or a group where you can get instruction. Start slow and be sure to get the green flag from your oncologist and your surgeon before starting an exercise regimen.

ROWING

While some exercises are solo in nature, rowing can be done on a team or solo. In fact, one of the most "club sports" supporting breast cancer patients has been rowing in the past several years. Breast cancer survivors around the country are joining dragon boat racing, which is an ancient Chinese water sport. Dragon boating is a vehicle for improving women's wellness and posttreatment quality of life. Rowing is an exercise that either requires the use of a rowing machine or an actual boat in an open body of water. It is an excellent aerobic exercise that works both the lower and upper body, thus is aerobic and strength training while being low impact in nature.

Rowing has many benefits as an exercise for cancer patients, ranging from physical to mental. Some benefits of rowing include

- Improved emotions due to increased production of endorphins (feel-good hormones) from exercise
- Significantly increased quality of life through team interactions and increased sense of community
- Maintenance of healthy body weight

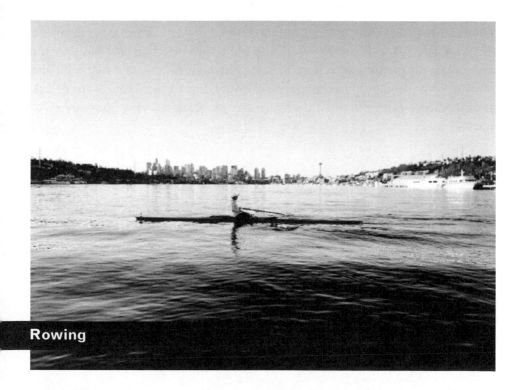

Rowing

- Efficient cardiac workout and strengthening for a healthy heart and lungs
- Full body muscular workout which increases flexibility and increases range of motion
- Is a nonimpact sport which is not hard on the joints
- Improved immune system and also memory

Like resistance training, the movement in rowing is repetitive and resistance can vary.

Using a Rowing Machine

If you have never used a rowing machine before, first go to a gym where you can get instruction on proper technique. Solo rowing is a very meditative exercise. Rowing and otherexercise machines can be purchased for home use.

Joining a Rowing Team

There are rowing teams throughout the United States. As mentioned earlier, there are also teams of survivors. These teams are beneficial for patients for the social and positive effects of moving through cancer as a team. Teams meet to row, frequently in the morning hours. Find a local row team or ask at your cancer center to see if there are any associated teams. Remember to start slow.

DANCING

According to the American Cancer Society, dance therapy is a physical activity which is beneficial for cancer patients. The physical effects are good, but the mental effects of dancing are outstanding for breast cancer patients. Many of the benefits involve the direct effect of increasing endorphin levels in the brain, which makes one feel comfortable and secure. In addition, dance therapy is aerobic and a weight-bearing exercise. You can join a dance therapy group or hire a professional dance therapist to guide your dancing individually, or you can simply turn on a couple of your favorite songs and start moving.

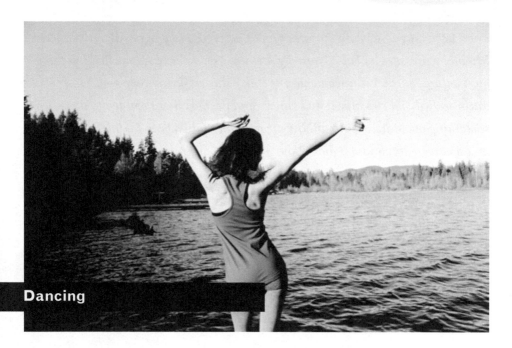

Dancing

Dance therapy has many benefits for breast cancer patients:

- Promotes healthy weight
- Strengthens muscles and bones
- Enhances the area of the brain that generally degenerates with age
- Improves balance
- Decreases anxiety

Wear comfortable clothing and find a place that you feel wholly uninhibited. Turn on your music and move however you feel you would like to. Note how your body feels. Is there any tightness or restrictions in your body? Do you have inhibitions or guarded movement? People engaging in dance therapy often keep a journal to write down and keep track of their feelings and physical manifestations. Like the recommendations for overall aerobic exercise, if dancing is your primary form of exercise, try to do it for 30 minutes four to five times a week.

RESOURCE

https://adta.org/

I had been diagnosed with diabetes type II before I was diagnosed with cancer. My blood pressure had also started going up. I was placed on medication for both before cancer. I learned about the link between poorer outcomes with uncontrolled diabetes type II and cancer and decided that I wanted to do something about it, and also all the medication that I'd been taking. While food and diet were important, I didn't know how important exercise was, resistance training, and aerobic exercise was to reversing it. I don't mind exercise, I just needed to make time for it. I needed to understand how important it was. Like Dr. Price said, it needs to be considered a medical prescription that happens every day. I feel great now. My blood sugar levels are controlled, and I check them daily, and my blood pressure is good.

—K.K.

CHAPTER 5

Finding Emotional Balance: Mind–Body Therapies for Patients With Breast Cancer

Your inner strength is your outer foundation.

—*Alan Rufus*

A diagnosis of cancer, and then the subsequent fast-paced movement into treatment, can be very traumatic. Patients often feel out of control, ungrounded, and have no idea where to begin to find their center. Depression and anxiety are common. These can significantly reduce quality of life. In addition, immune function can be affected by the production of stress hormones leading to less optimal outcomes.

There are several therapies that breast cancer patients can use to restore or balance emotional well-being. Each is slightly different and having different appeals. Some are done in groups, others solo; some involve art, others meditation. Whatever your preference, I highly recommend including one or more of these practices as part of your overall treatment toward remission. They and others are vital for optimal outcome.

YOGA

Yoga does not require fancy clothing or the ability to bend your leg behind your head to get started. To the contrary, in traditional practices yoga is noncompetitive, focusing on nonjudgment and starting where you are.

Yoga uses physical poses and breathing techniques to increase strength, flexibility, and well-being. It is both a physical exercise and meditative practice. Research in breast cancer patients has shown that yoga may be able to help

- Physical function
- Fatigue
- Stress and anxiety
- Sleep
- Quality of life

A study from the University of Texas MD Anderson Cancer Center investigated women with breast cancer and their ability to engage in their daily activities, general health, and fatigue. The study showed that all these activities improved with a yoga practice. Women in the yoga group had lower cortisol (the stress hormone). High levels of cortisol may be associated with poorer survival in women with breast cancer.

Another study from the Ohio State University found yoga lowered fatigue and reduced inflammation. In addition, according to the National Institutes of Health, evidence suggests yoga is helpful when used with conventional medical treatment to help relieve side effects of cancer treatment and other comorbidities like diabetes or arthritis. Sleep problems, depression, joint pain, and anxiety have all been reduced or resolved with yoga practice.

There are several different types of yoga, ranging from very gentle forms to very rigorous. I suggest finding a studio that offers hatha yoga, or that

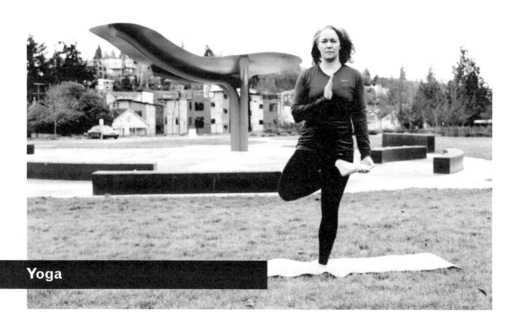

Yoga

offers classes for cancer patients. If you have never done yoga before, I recommend that you attend a class where you can learn correct form and be under the oversight of a skilled teacher. Proper form is essential for the practice to be effective and to avoid injury. Once you get more comfortable with the poses, you can practice them on your own or find an online video to use.

Yoga classes range in price from $15 to $25 per class. If you are a member of the YMCA, or are participating in the Livestrong program there, the classes are at no additional charge. Cancer support groups like Cancer Lifeline also offer low to no pay classes for patients and survivors. You should look for classes instructed by trained teachers. The classes are usually an hour long. Equipment that you might want to bring includes a yoga mat, but most studios have extra for attendees to use, along with blocks and other equipment to help make your class enjoyable.

Wear comfortable clothes to class that move and stretch. There is no need to go out and purchase expensive brands, unless you are a fashionista and it makes you feel better or more motivated.

RECOMMENDATIONS FOR FREQUENCY

Based on studies that I reviewed, I recommend that patients do yoga three times a week for 1-hour sessions. At this level is where most studies are seeing benefits, though practicing even once a week has positive effects.

RESOURCES

https://www.yogaalliance.org
https://www.youtube.com/watch?v=iY4CJK40kN0
https://www.youtube.com/watch?v=V1hbqmbw1xA
https://www.youtu.be/6LvVc74c1qo

GUIDED MEDITATION

Meditation can be defined as a practice of focusing one's mind to achieve mental clarity and emotional calm; or as I like to say, it helps quiet the normal stream of thoughts occupying your mind. It helps you to concentrate on the present moment rather than the past or future. Meditation is seen by many researchers as potentially one of the most effective forms of stress reduction. It has been shown to affect quality of life, immune

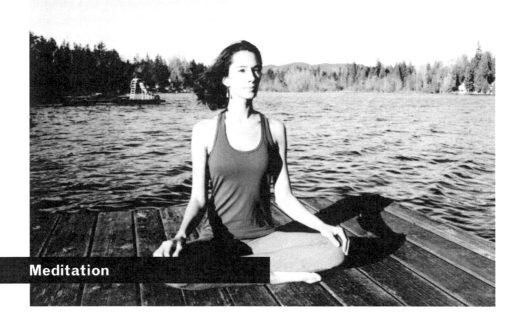

Meditation

function, restful sleep, energy, and improvement in mental health. For breast cancer patients, meditation helps deal with the anxiety and shock of diagnosis and fear of recurrence. More than 3,000 scientific studies have been conducted on the benefits of meditation and breast cancer. The results include positive outcomes for the treatment of depression and anxiety, and increases in concentration and memory. Studies have shown that meditation causes a shift and modulation of the immune system. The change involves T helper cells shifting from a general inflammatory state to one of an anti-inflammatory one.

Meditation is often referred to as a practice because to obtain mindfulness is easier said than done, but with time can be obtained. Sometimes meditation is called sitting, because one sits in a quiet location over a period, usually 10 to 20 minutes, clearing his or her mind. For many beginners, the most difficult part of the practice is to get their mind to be still, free of chatter. This difficulty is also the reason many are noncompliant. Because of this, I recommend guided meditation.

Guided meditation involves a trained guide or teacher, in person or via sound recording, video, or other audio–video media, helping one focus. It is one of the easiest ways to enter into a state of deep relaxation and inner stillness because your own chatter is displaced by the guide's voice. I often recommend guided meditation for people having sleep disturbances as well.

RESOURCES

I recommend using guided meditation in the morning after waking and in the evening right before bed. Here are some of my favorite resources

http://marc.ucla.edu/mindful-meditations

https://www.tarabrach.com/guided-meditations/

https://chopra.com/meditation

ART THERAPY

You do not have to be an artist to benefit from this very effective holistic therapy. In fact, counter to what it sounds like, completing an end product for show is not the point.

Art therapy uses the creative process to improve and enhance physical and emotional well-being. It provides a creative outlet for women with breast cancer and aids in reducing stress. Many cancer centers and hospitals provide this service to their patients. Individuals who most benefit are

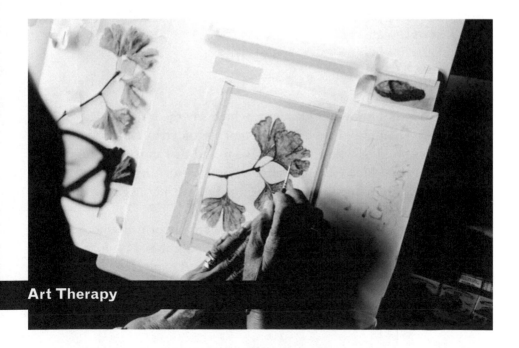

Art Therapy

those who are survivors of trauma and those with adverse physical health conditions like cancer.

According to one study, art therapy provoked brain changes linked with decreased stress in women. They experienced more cerebral blood flow and increased feelings of well-being. They also experienced less stress and anxiety, as well as increased emotional resiliency. A study of patients receiving radiation experienced mental, physical, and overall higher quality of life after five sessions of art therapy.

Some people may be intimidated by art therapy. It is important to be clear: art therapy is not about the end result, but it allows movement through emotions, emotions that patients might not even have the words for at the time. There is no judgment by the therapist.

Art therapy sessions are run by licensed counselors, who also have specialties and expertise in art therapy. It is important to find an art therapist who has training in working with breast cancer patients. Therapists will have all the equipment you will need; you will just have to get yourself to your session. If your clinic does not have an art therapist, you may find one by doing an online search for licensed art therapists.

RESOURCES

https://arttherapy.org/
https://www.nccata.org/

MUSIC THERAPY

Music therapy is a form of art therapy, which emerged in the 1940s. It uses music to effect a clinical change in clients and is guided by a trained therapist as they listen to music. Researchers have found that music modulates the activity of several limbic and paralimbic brain structures associated with pain, anxiety, and depression. It is effective in lowering negative emotions during administration of chemotherapy.

Patients are encouraged to communicate verbally or use other forms of communication like song writing, improvisation, musical performance, or even remaking a song to express themselves and explore their emotions. Those participating may play instruments, vocalize, or participate in music-guided imagery as well as just listen to music.

Several studies have documented the value of music therapy in reducing symptoms of anxiety, pain, fatigue, mood disturbances and improving ability to cope, social integration, and overall quality of life.

Like art therapy, many cancer centers offer music therapy. It is a cost-effective, noninvasive intervention that is free of side effects.

RESOURCES

https://www.musictherapy.org/
https://www.nccata.org/
https://www.wfmt.info/

QI GONG

Qi gong is a breath-focused, holistic system of coordinated body postures and movement, breathing, and meditation used for the purposes of health and as a martial arts training. It was developed a very long time ago in China. It is a gentle practice that can be done in a group or individually. It is well tolerated by people of all physical capacities.

In a study reported by the University of Texas MD Anderson Cancer Center published in 2013, investigators found that qi gong improved the quality of life of breast cancer patients.

Benefits for people with cancer include

- Mood improves and stress lessens while resiliency to adversity increases
- Fatigue lessens
- Inflammation decreases, including inflammatory markers
- Improved cognitive function
- Improved immune function as supported by studies
- Improved sleep

There are three main elements of qi gong exercise

- Slow fluid movements that mimic movements in nature. These exercises stretch and strengthen muscles.
- Deep breathing
- A meditative state of mind

Qi gong most recently has been found to have a significant effect on breast cancer patients and improving fatigue associated with treatment.

You might be surprised to find a number of studios that offer qi gong when you begin to look around. I would recommend going to a class that has an instructor, but qi gong can also be practiced safely by using an instructed video. Class prices are similar to yoga, ranging from $15 to $20. You need to wear loose-fitting, comfortable clothing, but nothing fancy.

RESOURCES

https://www.nqa.org/
https://www.qigonginstitute.org
https://www.youtube.com/watch?v=KcdcqW27RUs

I had never, ever seen myself as needing or using any kind of therapy. In our family you shut up, put up, and keep going. That wasn't working with cancer. I was having serious problems. The depression and anxiety were making it hard to do everything, work, sleep, interact with my family. I wasn't going to stick to something like meditation if I had to do it by myself, but I wasn't comfortable talking to someone one-on-one. I signed myself up for qi gong. My family questioned my choice, but I needed to do something. I loved it, and I loved how it made me feel. I still need to get to the point of speaking to someone, but the depression and anxiety have really decreased.

— L.B.

CHAPTER 6

Seeking Resiliency and Balance: Tying It All Together

My barn having burned down, I can now see the moon.

—*Mizuta Masahide*

This book presents a holistic and complementary plan for patients who have been diagnosed with breast cancer and who been treated with some form of conventional treatment. It provides a variety of safe and researched therapies that help decrease or prevent side effects associated with treatment and that address emotional well-being. Some suggestions are meant to be incorporated over a lifetime to help decrease risk of cancer recurrence and to maximize quality of life.

I have supplied you with quite a bit of information in a relatively small amount of space. Be cautious about thinking that you must incorporate everything at once. That is not how lifetime habits are formed and successful compliance is achieved. Small, consistent steps and a little self-understanding goes a long way, especially if these things are new to you.

I have had the honor of following breast cancer patients through their entire journey from diagnosis to remission and, therefore, have seen the journey and process of implementing holistic changes into their lives.

"Laurel" was one such patient. Laurel had been referred to me on the day of her diagnosis, and she immediately made an appointment. She was in shock, bewildered about the decisions she had to make about her treatment, and very anxious about the effects of treatment. Needless to say, she felt completely out of control.

Up to that point, Laurel had led what she considered a normal life. She ate out frequently, and her diet at home consisted mostly of easy to prepare or eat foods. She achieved 5,000 to 6,000 steps per day, but these were not related to consistent and focused aerobic or weight-bearing exercise.

Laurel reported that she had a large support network and community. Up to this point, she would split her time between her demanding job, raising her children, and being a key provider of support for that large support network she had.

Her initial worries with the diagnosis, surprisingly, were that her roles would be disrupted, and no one would be able to fill them. This is a quite frequent and normal response that is refocused or reprioritized with time and intervention.

As time passed, and as every patient knows, time during treatment seems to move quickly. Laurel and I developed a plan using many of the tools I have presented in this guide. We created a personalized, therapeutic diet, taking note of her treatment protocol, that also addressed preexisting conditions. She integrated more focused and consistent exercise during treatment as well.

Most surprising for both of us was her choice of art therapy. As she stated, she had shied away from art because she was not a particularly creative person and a perfectionist. Art therapy, she said, allowed her to express herself nonverbally with forms and colors. Images came first and were followed by articulated feelings. Her life shifted.

She began feeling a sense of control and began to look at all pieces of her life. What she would have called selfish behavior in the past for saying "no" became part of her daily routine. This became part of her time for taking care of herself. She began "weeding the garden," as she put it, removing draining relationships and activities that did not give her joy. She also created avenues for her children to be more independent and more helpful in the household. She continues using art therapy today to help her deal with the "monkey on her back," which is the potential of the cancer returning. Yet, with her holistic plan and sticking with her planned assessment schedule with her oncology team, she feels in control of the things that she can affect.

Most importantly, from all the holistic therapies that Laurel employed, dietary, exercise, and mind–body solutions, she developed greater resiliency and balance in her life. She was able to turn from despair to solutions. Something I wish for all readers and patients of this book to find.

APPENDIX

CANCER SUPPORT ORGANIZATIONS

Cancer organizations that can supply information on specific cancers and provide support during cancer treatment and beyond:

https://www.nationalbreastcancer.org/

http://www.abcf.org/

https://www.nationalbreastcancer.org/breast-cancer-support-groups

COUNSELING AND THERAPY ASSOCIATIONS

https://www.counseling.org/

https://ahha.org/

https://www.hypnosisalliance.com/iact/

EXERCISE ASSOCIATIONS AND INSTITUTIONS

Associations related to physical therapies, exercise, and other physical activities listed in the chapters of the book that are particularly helpful after cancer treatment:

http://www.internationalyogafederation.net/fiyorganizations.html

http://www.yogahealthfoundation.org/

https://www.nqa.org/

https://www.qigonginstitute.org/category/81/national-qigong-association

http://www.americantaichi.org/about.asp

http://www.taichifoundation.org/

http://americanmeditationsociety.org/

http://www.meditationinstructors.com/

INDEX